The Reset Factor

The Reset Factor

45 Days to Transforming Your Health by Repairing Your Gut

A STEP-BY-STEP GUIDE TO RECLAIMING THE BODY YOU WERE BORN TO LIVE IN.

By Dr. Mindy Pelz

Published by Reset Factor, LLC
364 E. Main St. Suite 549
Middletown, DE 19709

With the understanding that all individuals are complex and our health and fitness problems are unique the ideals, programs, plans, tools and suggestions in this book are not intended to replace the advice of trained medical professionals. All issues and questions regarding one's health care requires medical supervision. A physician should be consulted prior to adopting any program, plan, tool or idea described in this book. The contents of this book are based upon the opinion of the author. The author and publisher disclaim any liability arising directly or indirectly from the use of this book.

This book is not intended to make any recommendations related to getting on or off prescription or over-the-counter medication. If you face any current health concerns, or are currently taking medication, it is always recommended to seek the advice of your physician before starting a new nutrition or fitness program. While many of the testimonials shared in this book show patients becoming healthier and even getting off of drugs and medications, only medical doctors can prescribe drugs or tell you to reduce or stop taking a current prescription. This book's role is to make you aware of the hazards of poor lifestyle decisions while helping you to create better health habits resulting in improved innate healing of the body. As you heal using the tools, programs and plans in this book work with your medical doctor to reduce and hopefully eliminate the drugs you're on.

The information in this book is intended to be educational and should not replace consultation with a competent healthcare professional. The content of this book is intended to be used as an adjunct to responsible healthcare supervised by a healthcare professional. The author is not liable for any misuse of the material contained in this book.

First printing 2015
Printed in the United States of America
20 19 18 17 16 15   1 2 3 4 5

ISBN: 151929915X
ISBN 13: 9781519299154

reset

verb re·set \(,)rē-'set\

: to move (something) back to an original place or position

: to put (a broken bone) back in the correct position for healing

This book is dedicated to my dear friend Lani,
who never gave up on resetting her health
and inspiring others to do the same.

Contents

Preface

WHEN YOUR HEALTH GOES SOUTH, it turns your whole life upside down. I know—I've been there.

When I was 12 years old, I had one dream: to be a professional tennis player. For much of my youth, I spent hours training, traveling, and committing myself to being the best tennis player I could be. While other teens were hanging out on the beach, I was hitting balls on the tennis court. While most high schoolers were sleeping late on Saturday morning, I was on the tennis court before the sun was up. At a young age, I learned the power of sacrifice and commitment.

My senior year in high school, I was given the opportunity to join the women's tennis team at the University of Kansas and fight for a scholarship position. I was elated. It was a dream I had worked hard for—and I was ready for the challenge. Tennis is a sport that tests you physically and mentally: you have to train your body to endure heat, move your feet fast in all directions, last through long rallies, and have quick reflexes. More importantly, you have to train your mind to be patient and strategic, to never give up, to play each point one at a time, and to persist despite any obstacle that is put in your way. When I finally got the scholarship, I realized that there's no greater feeling than persevering through hard work and obstacles—and getting results for it.

Then, two years into my collegiate tennis career, my body began to break down. At nineteen years old, all the training had caught up with me; my body was tired. It started during one practice, when I noticed my shins were hurting. Within weeks, mild pain turned into chronic, severe, relentless pain. I was diagnosed with shin splints and told ice and ibuprofen would be the fix.

The ibuprofen solved the pain problem temporarily. Yet, like most injuries in the body, if you don't get to the cause of the injury, it will continue to get worse. That's exactly what happened. While I was taking large amounts of ibuprofen daily to manage the pain, the injury grew worse.

Every doctor I consulted gave me a stronger painkiller. Each time I tried the new painkiller, it felt like a miracle cure, yet weeks later it would stop working. At nineteen years old, I couldn't make it through my daily life without a painkiller. This went on for a year and a half.

Finally, an orthopedic surgeon was called in to evaluate me. He diagnosed me with *compartment syndrome,* a condition in the lower legs where the muscles are so swollen that the fascia surrounding them thickens and creates intense pressure in the lower leg "compartments." This condition creates a sharp stabbing pain that feels as if someone is shooting pellets into your calves. I was immediately scheduled for surgery.

Recovery was supposed to be quick—three months, tops. We were in the tennis off-season, so the plan was for me to have surgery in October and be back on the court training in December. But things didn't go as expected.

Once out of surgery, I was quickly put on more medications—stronger ones than those I had been taking for the past few years. And as I waited to get back on the courts, I quickly fell into the typical college life: poor diet, late nights, beer, pizza, and partying. I gained thirty pounds over a couple of months, and although my leg pain was improving, my health was at an all-time low. By Christmas, my body was so fatigued I couldn't get out of bed.

Watching my health spiral downward was one of the scariest and most frustrating experiences of my life. Bouncing from doctor to doctor looking for answers started to make me feel as if I were crazy. Luckily, one person was there to lift me up and keep me going: my mom.

When I went home over Christmas break, my mom could see that years of training, popping pain pills, and going through surgery had left my body in a massively fatigued state. Being the tenacious woman that she was, she quickly started searching for answers about chronic fatigue. Finally, with persistence, we found a top chronic fatigue doctor who happened to practice in our town. Our hope was restored.

Now, when you're a patient struggling with your health, your doctor quickly becomes the most important person in your life. He or she becomes your lifeline. You trust that your doctor will find the answer for you, wants you to get better, cares about you, and will give you a new direction. We want our doctors to have all the answers—to be superhuman.

But the day we walked into that doctor's office forever changed the way I look at the doctor-patient relationship. The doctor sat behind a large mahogany desk wearing a white coat. He was a bit intimidating, but for the most part, I was relieved by the way he looked because society had trained me to view anyone in a white coat as knowledgeable. He looked capable, smart, and resourceful.

Sadly, my opinion quickly changed. As my mom began to tell my story, the doctor looked disinterested, a little arrogant, as if we were somehow inconveniencing him with my story. He seemed more interested in writing me a prescription than in understanding how my health had broken down.

My mom's number-one concern was for him to give me a path to getting my body strong enough to get me back to school as quickly as possible. When she asked him how he could help me do this, he laughed with an arrogant smirk on his face and said, "Does she look like she can go back to school?" As if the idea that the body could heal quickly from such a condition as mine was too stupid even to consider.

He then proceeded to take out a long list of medications. He explained that some of these medications had worked on cases like mine but that chronic fatigue syndrome was not the same in every individual. His recommendation: start with the first one. If that didn't work, move to the next one, and so on and so forth. Within a year's time, he said, we would know which medication might help my chronic fatigue. In the meantime, his advice was to drop out of school and wait for one of the medications to work.

Now let's stop and review what I had been through in the years prior to my chronic fatigue: daily pain medication, poor diet, improper sleep, pushing myself physically, stress, late nights drinking, surgery, increasingly strong pain medications, and eventually even multiple medications. Another medication was not going to be my answer, and wasting a year of my life hoping a new medication would solve my problem was not my definition of a plan. I had destroyed my body from the inside—and there wasn't one chemical that was going to bring me back to normal again.

What I needed was a reset. A do-over. I needed to repair the damage I had done.

I needed a doctor who could see the big picture—what systems were broken inside me. I needed a doctor who cared about finding the *cause* of my health problems. I needed a doctor who believed in me and who could teach me a path to rebuilding my body back to its original design. And I had no idea where to turn.

But my mom did. She found several doctors who believed in me and the power of my body to heal, and the month that followed consisted of visits to some of them—health practitioners who could actually help me.

The first doctor I saw was a holistic MD who immediately taught me how to stop putting toxins into my body. He knew that 80 percent of the immune system lived in the gut, and that if I was to heal, I would need to repair that system first. He put me on a healing diet and restricted me from eating any foods that would destroy my gut and suppress my immune system. He then prescribed a protocol of supplements to repair the damage that years of medications and poor diet had done to my body. Vitamin C drips, B12 shots, high doses of probiotics, enzymes, and anti-fungal supplements became a weekly regimen for me.

We then sought out the expertise of a "corrective" chiropractor to help open up the flow of information coming out of my brain and restore the function of my nervous system. This sped up my healing and had me sleeping and thinking better. Then we found an expert in stress management, who taught me techniques for managing stress and showed me how to harness the power of using my mind to visualize the body healing.

It was a powerful team approach to regaining my health—one that was focused on repairing the damage that my lifestyle, medications, and stress had done, giving my body back its power and giving it a fighting chance to heal itself.

THE POWER TO HEAL

No one ever teaches us that our bodies are powerful healers. From the day we're born, we're taught to put things from the outside into us to heal. Parents are told that their child's immune system is weak and that they need to keep their child away from germs, vaccinate him because he's too weak to fight bacteria on his own, medicate him when he has symptoms—and if necessary, do surgery to repair something inside him that's malfunctioning. This outside-in approach to taking care of our health gives all the power to the medication and the doctor. And it almost destroyed my life. But after three weeks on my natural protocols, my energy started coming back. I quickly dropped the thirty pounds I had gained. I began sleeping better. I started feeling more hopeful and positive about my future. I felt as if someone had turned on a light switch inside me, as I was now healing from the inside out.

A month after I walked into the chronic fatigue specialist's office, I was on a plane heading back to college. Six weeks after that, I was on the tennis court, energized and pain-free. In the months that followed, my recovery gained momentum. Each day I felt stronger and stronger. The prognosis by one of our country's finest doctors for the time it would take to treat and heal the symptom of fatigue was at least a year. Yet I experienced that repairing the cause of my fatigue took a fraction of that time. And to this day, I have never struggled with that level of fatigue again.

That experience changed my life forever. What I learned from the team of doctors who helped me was that *our bodies are incredible healers*. The doctors took the time to teach me how my body works and where the breakdowns in my health were—and then they gave me the tools to fix those breakdowns. Those doctors believed in me and my power to heal. Their knowledge, belief, and commitment to help me inspired me to go to chiropractic school. It motivated me to turn around and teach others what I had learned. It resulted in the creation of the 45-Day Reset, which is the heart of my work and this book.

For the past twenty years, I've been in the trenches of health with my patients. I call it "the trenches of health" because we live in a time when our bodies are constantly being bombarded in a way that creates physical, emotional, and chemical traumas. Our bodies are living in a war zone every day.

No organ in the body is more vulnerable to these traumas than our gastrointestinal system. Much like what happened to me, many people are experiencing breakdowns in their health. Yet we have a health care system built on treating the symptoms of these breakdowns, not getting to the cause of them. In fact, in many cases, the medical responses to symptoms are causing more damage to the gut, leaving the body worse off than it was before. As a result, I have dedicated my life to helping people understand the cause of their poor health and giving them the tools never to let their health break down again.

This book is about giving you the same understanding, teaching you how your body works and how to repair your gut, and handing you the tools to be the boss of your own health care. It's my hope that you will find the answers to your health challenges herein. But understand, this is not a book about curing your disease. It's about making you strong again. It's about restoring that amazing healing power you were born with. When you start to build your body strong from the inside out, miracles happen.

I'm excited to be on this journey with you!

Acknowledgments

I HAD NO IDEA THE day I left the chronic fatigue specialist's office, feeling hopeless and frustrated, that my health breakdown would launch a lifetime of passion and commitment to help people find real solutions to their health problems—and that it would result in my writing this book.

I have many people to thank for the role they played in this creation. First, this book would have never happened without the courage and commitment of the amazing group of patients I have had the pleasure of helping over the years. You all inspire me and ignite a fire in me to help find you the best health solutions available. Thank you for letting me walk alongside you in your journey back to health and for having the strength and commitment to keep making your health a priority.

To Lani, to whom this book is dedicated, I wish the 30-year-old version of you had access to the information on these pages. I have no doubt that if you had, you would be with us today. Thank you for taking your personal health crisis and using it as a tool to inspire others to commit to their health. You opened your heart to all of us and let us walk your journey of cancer with you—and even up till the day you died, you worked to educate others on how not to end up with the disease path you had been given. I miss you every day and will spend the rest of my life carrying your mission forward.

I am forever grateful to the mentors in my life who paved a path for me. My first health mentor was my mom. I feel so blessed to have been born to a woman who made health a priority from the day I was born. My first chiropractor, Dr. Roger Akers, DC, taught me how powerful a chiropractic adjustment can be to the human body. Dr. Luc DeShepperd, MD, proved to me that if you change your diet, you'll change your health. Drs. Ron and Mary Oberstein, DC, modeled for me how rewarding a life of service and purpose can be. And finally, Dr. Charles Majors, DC, showed me that anything is possible when you pair an unwavering belief with a ridiculous amount of action.

I also know that the journey I have been on with my patients would have never been possible without the amazing staff I have had the pleasure of working with over the years. Every one of you brought to our patients a healing energy and commitment for which I am eternally grateful.

For years, people kept telling me to put the work I do in my office into a book. When I finally committed to doing that, I started and stopped many times. Finally, it was the encouragement of the Reset Factor team, Madeleine and Alex, who gave me the vision to see how this information could transform lives.

My editor, Jennifer Read Hawthorne, had the daunting task of taking my words and turning them into magic. There is absolutely no way this book would have been published without her wisdom, patience, and ability to pull information out of my brain and put it onto these pages in a way that people could understand easily and apply effortlessly. I am so grateful for her guidance and support.

To my kids, Bodhi and Paxton, I know having a mother who is obsessed with her work is not always easy. Searching for answers to people's health crises has required me to fly all over the country to attend seminars and learn from experts, and it has constantly kept me on the phone in conference calls or on my computer writing. It has killed me every time I missed one of your special events, soccer games, vaulting competitions, or school outings. Thank you for understanding and supporting me, and for always cheering me on. I am so proud of you and the amazing people you have become.

Last, to my husband, Sequoia, you are my rock. Thank you for being my number-one fan. You never stop believing in me, cheering me on, and encouraging me to keep moving forward. You never complain about having to take on more work at home or about driving the kids to one more event while I put in extra time working. You are always willing to be the guinea pig for any new health idea I want to try out. Without your support and love, this book would have never happened. Thank you for loving me so much and walking this crazy path of service with me.

Part 1

~&

Why We Need to Reset Our Bodies

Introduction

THERE ARE NO COINCIDENCES IN life. You picked up this book for a reason. And no matter where you are with your health today, you can change it. I promise. I watch it happen all the time.

The information on the following pages is an accumulation of over twenty years experience helping thousands of people reset their health—and I want to help you reset yours. Why? Because our current approach to health *is not working!* We need to create a health care system that is dedicated to rebuilding the body, not just treating symptoms. We need doctors who see people, not conditions—unlike the chronic fatigue specialist I met with on that winter day who could see only my syndrome, not me. He didn't stop to ask why I was so tired or where my body had broken down or what was causing the breakdown. All he could see was a symptom, a diagnosis, and its solution: drugs.

Yet these are some of the most important questions you can ask when you're sick: Why is my body feeling this way? What system or systems are not working right? What aspect of my body is so depleted that it's causing me to feel like this?

After years of coaching people to better health, I've discovered that most people have a desire to be healthy—but they simply don't have a clear path to accomplishing their desire. We need a user's manual for this miraculous body we live in.

It's time to take back your health! It's time to understand that the body you have been given has an incredible ability to heal and perform at whatever level you desire.

It's time for a reset.

Modern Living and the Rise of Chronic Disease

The health of our communities is at a critical point. Obesity, heart attacks, diabetes, and cancer are at an all-time high. Seventy percent of Americans are on a medication.[1] The United States Centers for Disease Control and Prevention (CDC) 2009 statistics on deaths due to medications showed that for the first time ever in the United States, more people were killed by drugs (over-the-counter and prescription) than motor vehicle accidents.[2] Drug fatalities more than doubled among teens and young adults between 2000 and 2008,[3] and they more than tripled among people aged fifty to sixty-nine. These drug-induced fatalities are not being driven by illegal street drugs; the analysis found that the most commonly abused prescription drugs—like OxyContin, Vicodin, Xanax, and Soma—now cause more deaths than heroin and cocaine combined. Tylenol is the top offender on the list of common drugs that people die from due to an overdose.

In 2009, concerned about the growing toxic load on our children, the Environmental Working Group (EWG) did a study measuring the number of chemicals present in newborn babies. They took ten Americans from different parts of the country and measured the chemicals and pollutants in their blood. These ten children had one thing in common: it was their first day of life. The results were astonishing. An average of

---

1 "Nearly 7 in 10 Americans Are on Prescription Drugs," *Science Daily,* June 19, 2013, http://www.sciencedaily.com/releases/2013/06/130619132352.htm.
2 Centers for Disease Control and Prevention, "Drug Poisoning Deaths in the United States, 1980–2008," NCHS Data Brief, no. 81 (December 2011), http://www.cdc.gov/nchs/data/databriefs/db81.htm.
3 Centers for Disease Control and Prevention, "Injury Prevention & Control: Prescription Drug Overdose," http://www.cdc.gov/drugoverdose/

200 industrial chemicals and pollutants (out of 413 tested) were found in the umbilical cord blood of these ten babies born in August and September of 2004 in US hospitals. The umbilical cord blood contained pesticides; personal care product ingredients; and toxins from burning coal, gasoline, and garbage.

Of the 287 total chemicals and pollutants detected in the umbilical cord blood, scientists have shown that 134 cause cancer, 158 are toxic to the brain and nervous system, 186 cause infertility, and 151 cause birth defects or abnormal development. Shockingly, 212 of the industrial chemicals and pesticides found were banned over thirty years ago.

How could this have happened? Why is no one talking about it? How are these chemicals getting into our systems? If they're present in our environment, food, water, and medications, we need to start asking ourselves how we can take personal action to minimize the damage they're having on our bodies.

Clearly, our children are suffering the most from this toxic overload. One in every sixty-eight children is diagnosed with autism spectrum disorders.[4] These numbers, compiled in 2010 by the CDC, show that autism spectrum disorders have more than doubled since the CDC's 2002 survey. What troubles specialists researching autism spectrum disorders is that this surge, which has continued unabated year after year, exhibits only minimal variation among races, regions, and socioeconomic groups. Autism has gone up in every group, every way you slice it. Something is affecting the population—the whole population.

Cancer has now become the number-one killer of our children ages five to fourteen, six being the average age for a cancer diagnosis. Studies of possible environmental risk factors include prenatal exposure to cancer-causing chemicals and pesticides, plus childhood exposure to common infectious agents (including vaccines).

---

4 Centers for Disease Control and Prevention, "Prevalence of Autism Spectrum Disorder Among Children Aged 8 Years," *Morbidity and Mortality Weekly Report* 63 (SS02), March 28, 2014, http://www.cdc.gov/mmwr/preview/mmwrhtml/ss6302a1.htm.

The medicines we have relied on for years to cure us are now failing. Antibiotics provide a good example of this. The massive amount of antibiotic use in our country has turned the bacterial world into the domain of superbugs that are only getting stronger. Antibiotics are not as effective as they were years ago.

I recently had a nutrition consultation with an eighteen-year-old college student who was concerned with her worsening skin problems and depleted immune system. She had seen several doctors whose only solution was more medication. Nothing was helping and the doctors were out of answers for her. She came to me frustrated and losing hope she would ever have clear skin again.

When I went through her health history, I learned she had been on over twenty rounds of antibiotics. That is more than most people will take in their lifetime—and she was eighteen. Antibiotics are known to kill all the bad *and* good bacteria in our guts, leaving the gut in a very vulnerable state. When our guts are out of balance, our whole body can break down.

The young woman's skin and poor health were indicators of the beginning of this breakdown. The solution for this young woman was not more toxins—it was to repair her gut and build her body strong again, from the inside out.

Food allergies constitute another growing epidemic. One out of thirteen children now has a food allergy.[5] The number of people suffering from food allergies has more than doubled in the past decade, and hospitalizations for food allergies increased by 500 percent from 1990 to 2006. In the United States, about ninety thousand people visit the emergency room each year due to food allergies.

Often, a person is allergic to a commonly eaten food. Most people are surprised to learn that the foods they love and eat every day are often the ones they are allergic too. (I'll walk you through these foods in Chapter 2.) Schools are now having to go to great lengths to

5 "Facts and Statistics," Food Allergy Research & Education website, accessed October 30, 2015, https://www.foodallergy.org/facts-and-stats/

accommodate for these allergies, as the list of children with deadly allergies is growing. Most elementary school teachers are now well versed in how to use an EpiPen® Auto-Injector. Whole sections of lunch tables are quarantined for allergen-free lunches—a practice rarely seen decades ago.

What would make our children react so much to foods? If 80 percent of our immune system comes from our gut, is it possible that damage to the gut suppresses our immune system and makes us more susceptible to allergies? Maybe all the harmful chemicals we're exposed to—the same ones the EWG found in newborn babies—are beginning to weaken our digestive system. Is it a coincidence that food allergies are becoming more common, or is it that our bodies are trying to adapt to our new chemical environment?

Asthma is also on the rise. The prevalence of asthma has been increasing since the early 1980s across all age, sex, and racial groups. Asthma accounts for almost 2 million emergency room visits, 14 million doctor visits, and 439,000 hospitalizations each year. More than 3,600 deaths are attributed to asthma each year—that's nine Americans each day. Something has to be triggering this increase.

Numerous children have come to me with chronic asthma problems. Most of them are on inhalers, which are filled with toxic chemicals that destroy healthy tissues—chemicals like corticosteroids. One young girl in particular was greatly affected by her debilitating asthma—so much so that it was causing her to miss out on her childhood. She was constantly sick and wheezy, and many allergens in the air would set off her asthma. When her medical doctor measured her lung capacity, the doctor found she was spending much of her days low on oxygen. The young girl was prescribed inhalers to be used for the rest of her life.

When she came to me, her condition was beginning to worsen. Her parents were looking for a solution other than chronic medications. We implemented a plan to strengthen her gut and stop the breakdowns in her body—and within six months she was off all inhalers. Her medical doctor re-measured her lung capacity and declared her asthma-free.

What is causing so many people to have a weakened immune system? How can so many people be susceptible to food allergies? What would cause so many people to get asthma?

More and more families are seeing breakdowns in their health. No one is immune from the growing epidemic of chronic diseases and increasing toxic loads. Think back to when you were a child. The majority of people with cardiovascular diseases, stroke, and cancer were elderly. In recent years, however, the majority of people suffering from serious illnesses have been the young-to-middle-aged-adult population.

This crazy-busy lifestyle is destroying our health. Look around you. Hormone problems, digestive complaints, low energy, unexplained weight gain, and chronic pain have all become accepted norms. And unfortunately, our culture has come to accept that having a high-stress lifestyle means having a low level of health.

It's time to do health differently.

HOW WE MANAGE OUR HEALTH TODAY

Think about the last time you were not feeling well. What was the first thing you did to relieve your pain? For most of us, the answer is to take a pill—that's what we've been taught to do. Yet if chemicals in our foods and environment are destroying our health, can a chemical in a pill restore our health?

Let's look at what your symptoms are telling you. Symptoms are how your body tells your brain that something is wrong. They're your body's dashboard; when a dashboard light turns on, what is your car telling you to do? Stop and get your engine looked at, right? Symptoms are the same thing. Symptoms are how your body talks to your brain, giving you an assessment of what's happening "under the hood." Back pain, headaches, digestive issues, allergies, fatigue, cloudy thinking, depression, and unexplained weight gain are all signals from your body that something is breaking down.

A 40-year-old woman came to my office this year with such severe low back pain that she couldn't even put on her own underwear. She is a professional woman with a family and a very successful job, and she spent the past decade putting her family and career ahead of her health. She managed her pain with daily medication and grit, and she came to accept her pain as part of the aging process.

But after years of popping pain pills and accepting this low standard of health, she decided to sit down with me and create a plan to build her body strong again. My tests found that years of medications and poor lifestyle had destroyed her gut. Her bad bacteria counts were some of the highest I had ever seen.

I immediately put her on the 15-Day GI and Liver Detox (the first part of the 45-Day Reset) to repair her gut and liver. Within three days, miracles began to happen. First, her mobility came back. Then, her pain started to diminish. And finally, her stomach began to flatten. By the end of the fifteen days, she was full of energy, she had lost seven pounds, her pain was 70 percent gone, and her stomach was flattening out.

It's a growing challenge, the fact that we've been taught to take a pill when symptoms appear. This mindset toward our health is why the United States is one of the sickest countries in the developed world despite spending the most money per capita. We have a medicine mindset. We have more faith in a pill than in the healing power of our own bodies. Taking a pill is easy—it requires no personal responsibility. It means we don't have to change the foods we eat, exercise more, or stress less.

But the bad news is this: taking a pill is not a permanent solution to our health problems. This is why many people find their list of medications growing every year. This is why we are getting sicker and sicker despite being on the latest and greatest drug. We are only masking symptoms, not addressing causes.

The good news is that many people are starting to wake up to the fact that there is another way to take care of their health. People are tired of all the side effects medications create. Many are searching for new answers to their health problems. Once you make the decision to heal yourself from the inside out, you feel empowered. You are now the one in control of your health.

The challenge many people find is that there is an overwhelming amount of information on nutrition, exercise, and stress available today. If you made a decision to start a journey toward true health and you googled "nutrition," the amount of information you'd have access to would be overwhelming. You would not find a clear path to understanding what foods you need to eat.

HOW THE RESET PROGRAM WAS BORN

Depressed yet? Don't be. There is hope. What most people haven't realized is that no matter where you are with your health—or lack of it—you can reset the healing power of your body. That is why the program I've created is called the 45-Day Reset. It's the one part of health that people forget to factor in. It's *never* too late to reset your health. Recognize that you have *power within you that wants to heal.* No matter how bad your health problems are, don't forget to factor in that *your body is craving a reset*—and once you give it one, healing can happen.

The 45-Day Reset is a result of over twenty years working with thousands of people needing a new solution to their health crises. The program is based on hard scientific research and years of real-world success with my patients.

Many leading health experts now know what foods your body needs to thrive, what toxins break down your immune system, how the gut gets out of balance, and how this creates a spiral of poor health. We can clearly see why chronic pain can come from a broken digestive system. And we now know that weight problems are not a calorie issue but a hormonal one.

The tools and research are summarized in this book for you. In this program, I'll give you a proven path to rebuilding your body back to the way it was designed to be. You'll learn how to repair the damage that years of stressful toxic living may have done to you. You'll be given the tools to bring your body back into balance and have it performing at the level where it was meant to be. A Reset is what you need to regain your health and be disease-free for the rest of your life.

Once done, you will lose weight without having to starve yourself or work extra hard at the gym. Risks for diseases will also decrease, allowing you to live a fuller, happier, healthier life. You'll get to enjoy more things in life because your mind and body are able to feel more, focus on important things, and achieve more.

This is the 45-Day Reset, *your step-by-step path to a higher level of health.*

How to Use This Book

The book is divided into three parts. Part 1 (the Introduction and Chapter 1) focuses on how most of us are approaching our health—an approach that is broken. Understanding that you can apply a different approach is pivotal to your success with the 45-Day Reset.

Part 2 (Chapters 2 through 7) is the nuts and bolts of how your body functions and why it breaks down. I go in depth on how breakdowns happen and the science of how we can fix the underlying problems that cause breakdowns. If you understand why your health got off track, then you're less likely to create the same problems again.

Part 3 (Chapters 8 through 11) contains the toolset, the details of the 45-Day Reset Program. I will talk about how to set yourself up to make sure you succeed with the program. Next, I cover the nine profound "reset truths of health" that will help you understand how to make health a lifestyle change—not just some fleeting diet that doesn't work.

So let's start at the beginning: let's take a closer look at how best you can approach your health so that you can quickly put yourself back on the path to a new and extraordinary life.

CHAPTER 1

How to Feel Twenty Again

A healthy outside starts from the inside.

—Robert Urich

WE HUMANS ARE SELF-HEALING MACHINES. When you cut your finger, what does your body do? It immediately starts a clotting process to stop the bleeding. It creates collagen to repair the broken skin. And we don't even have to think about it. We put a Band-Aid on it and just know that it will heal.

The same thing happens when we get an infection. Our body produces a cough or fever to destroy the harmful intruder. Again, no conscious thought is needed; our body just does it innately.

This level of repair is happening in your body all day long. Your digestion, your metabolism, your hormones, your immune system—they all have the capability to self- regulate. So if you've hit a place with your health where you feel stuck—you're gaining weight, you're losing energy, or you're feeling depressed—I have great news for you: your body wants to repair itself. You can feel twenty again!

The trick is understanding why your body broke down in the first place. So in the next few chapters, I'll help you understand *how* your body works, *why* it breaks down, and *what* you can do about it. You need a proven path to regaining your health—not another broken promise. A path that will have you feeling twenty again.

In this chapter, we'll explore how the 45-Day Reset works with your body's own intelligence, what the body's original design looks like, why we need to reset our bodies, the limitations of a symptom-based approach to health, and how the 45-Day Reset works.

Healing from the Inside Out

The 45-Day Reset helps your body heal from the inside out. It brings your body back to its original design. It turns on your self-correcting, self-regulating healing power. While many programs offer you quick fixes without lasting results, the 45-Day Reset reprograms the body back to its original unspoiled and undisturbed state.

Every process within the body is perfectly designed to supply the body's particular needs. Every tissue is perfectly designed to carry out its special functions. Every organ is designed to complement the function of other tissues. All systems work hand in hand to make sure that the body meets its daily nutrient and energy requirements, as well as effectively removing any waste and toxins that result from these processes.

In this day and age, key systems of the body are breaking down. Toxins are bombarding you every second, causing your body to work overtime. They're shutting down the self-repair mechanisms of your body. This is why a reset is crucially important.

Your Body's Original Design

Did you miss reading the user's manual that came with your body? Well, don't feel bad—most people did. Before we get into the nuts and bolts of the 45-Day Reset, let's take a moment to help you understand how your body was designed to work. Think of this book as your user's manual. It will teach you how to treat your body the way it wants to be treated.

First, think of all your cells like pieces of a puzzle that go together to create a masterful picture. If you're missing one piece, the whole picture is thrown off.

We have over seventy-two trillion cells in our body. Every single cell in the body functions in coordination with adjacent cells. Each small cell function plays an important role in the body's overall functioning.

For example, the cells in your digestive system need to be in perfect balance in order for the neurotransmitters in your brain to work properly (more on this in Chapter 3). When we experience conditions in our brain like depression or mental fogginess, we immediately assume the problem must lie in the brain. We don't go digging for where the depleted chemicals related to these problems are made. We just see the deficiency and replenish those depleted chemicals through synthetic medications. We forget the interconnectedness of every cell of our body.

I had a 45-year-old woman come to me complaining of depression and lack of mental clarity. She often felt teary and hopeless for no reason. Normally an optimistic person, she felt as if someone else were controlling her thoughts. Her life was great; she had no reason to be sad. Her doctor recommended antidepressants, but she didn't want another medication.

Knowing that the hormones that make us happy are made in the gut, I recommended that we begin by repairing that organ and waiting to see what would happen. Within two weeks on the 15-Day GI and Liver Detox, her moods improved and her mental clarity was restored. The body didn't need another toxin—it needed her to reset the malfunction.

WHY RESET?

In his book *Clean,* Dr. Alejandro Junger writes: "The time has come when we are waking up to an alarming truth. We are killing ourselves with the same chemicals we invented to make our lives easier."

Whether you are aware of it or not, we don't live in the same world we grew up in. Our world is a hundred times more toxic. As I pointed out in the introduction, toxins are everywhere! Our food, water, air, household cleaners, and beauty products are more toxic than ever before. No one is immune from the growing number of toxins we are exposed to.

One of the systems vulnerable to these toxins is our digestive system. Foods made from genetically modified organisms (GMOs), partially hydrogenated oils, and man-made chemicals are killing what is called the microbiome of our gastrointestinal systems. The *microbiome* is the community of bacteria, good and bad, that live mostly in your gut.

The human body contains over ten times more microbial cells than human cells. This eclectic grouping of bacteria is said to account for 1 to 3 percent of our total body mass and weighs approximately two to three pounds. That means that every time you step on the scale, two to three pounds of the number you see there is bacteria. This complex group of bacteria has to be in perfect balance in order for your immune system, brain, and hormones to function properly.

One of the reasons people are more obese, more depressed, and more fatigued than ever before is because of the damage to this microbiome that is being caused by toxins in people's bodies. To protect itself from toxins, your digestive system inflames. This can leave you feeling constantly bloated, fatigued, lacking in mental clarity, and in pain.

The brain is also affected by this change in the microbiome. Neurotransmitters that are made in the gut become depleted, leaving the brain without the key amino acids that it needs to function normally. B vitamins are also made in the gut, and without the proper balance of bacteria, they too become depleted, leaving many people fatigued and weak.

Your immune system is greatly affected by your bacterial balance as well. If your microbiome is out of balance, your immune system will be out of balance. Dr. Joseph Mercola writes that increasing cancer rates have clear links to the toxins that are killing the healthy bacteria in the gut, destroying our body's immune capability to fight cancer.

For most people, these toxins keep coming. I see them every day in my practice: people whose bodies have started to break down and who are in desperate need of a repair. Their bodies never get a rest.

THE PROBLEM WITH OUR SYMPTOM-BASED APPROACH TO HEALTH

Symptoms related to damaged organs do not develop overnight, nor in days or weeks. It takes years of an unhealthy lifestyle, exposure to toxins, and neglect of the body before symptoms appear. Most of us start life off at 100 percent function, all systems functioning smoothly. At this point, the body is like a brand-new engine with all its gears, pistons, and other parts sparkling, shiny, and well oiled.

As the body starts to become exposed to toxins—from food, water, air, and other environmental conditions—damage slowly starts to add up. At first, there are no outward signs that something bad is happening in the body. This is because the body has an integral backup plan in case some parts of its systems can't function well.

When damage to the cells of the body continue and overall function diminishes to 60 percent, the body's compensatory mechanism can no longer take over the function of the damaged tissues. In my experience, this is when a person starts to feel symptoms such as pain, fatigue, weight gain, and depression.

Since we have been taught to take care of our bodies only when we "feel" a breakdown, many people believe that their health problem started when their symptoms began. Nothing could be further from the truth. It takes years for the damage from toxic living to produce a symptom.

Cancer is a great example of this. William Li, MD, President and Medical Director of the Angiogenesis Foundation, has given a TED Talk on how to eat to starve cancer; he talks about how most of us have anywhere from one to ten thousand cancer cells inside us right now. Hopefully, you have a strong immune system that will identify and destroy those cells. But what if your immune system were weakened? What if the cancer cells continued to multiply? When would you notice it? Unfortunately, it takes millions of cancer cells and, in some cases, close to seven years for cancer to grow to the point that it can be identified with diagnostic testing. The scary thing is that even at that point, you may not have a symptom.

HOW THE 45-DAY RESET FACTOR PROGRAM WORKS

Convinced yet that your efforts are best spent repairing breakdowns in your body instead of masking symptoms? The 45-Day Reset is designed specifically to repair your damaged gut, reset your metabolism, improve your mental clarity, strengthen your immune system, detoxify your liver, increase your happiness, and give you an abundance of energy. No joke. You can live in a body that feels that great and functions that well.

The 45-Day Reset lasts for 45 days and consists of two phases. The initial phase is the 15-Day GI and Liver Detox to help you reset your liver, digestion, and hormones. In this phase, you'll eliminate foods that are interfering with your body's original design, giving your digestion a break—much like the homeopathic doctor did for me in my chronic-fatigue state.

You'll also begin to add back in good bacteria, enzymes, and amino acids to repair your microbiome. You'll flood your liver with nutrients that are essential to its ability to effectively detoxify.

Last, you'll begin the process of balancing your hormones. Hormone receptor sites for insulin, cortisol, and leptin that have been clogged with toxins will become unblocked, allowing your body to finally be able to balance these crucial hormones. This turns on the fat-burning switch and tells your body to use energy from fat. I often see people lose anywhere from five to ten pounds during this crucial detoxifying phase.

The second phase is the 30-Day Habit Reset. This retraining phase will help you reset your taste buds, daily habits, and mindset about health while continuing to repair organs that have been damaged from toxic living. Most people experience profound weight loss during this phase. Because your hormones will be balancing out, you'll notice that your hunger is gone and your energy is high. During this second phase, your body will begin to crave health more than it does the habits that have been destroying it.

Before you start the initial phase of the program, I'll outline the "reset rules" of health. These rules will give you the necessary tools to keep weight off for good and have your body functioning at the highest levels possible for years to come.

Depending on where your health is when you start, the first three to five days of the detox are typically the hardest. Most people start off the first day enthusiastic and finish that day with an acute awareness of just how strong their cravings are. Usually, the second and third days are when the withdrawal from sugar kicks in and the brain begins to try to talk you out of this new way of eating. By the fourth and fifth day, fatigue, cloudy thinking, and crankiness can be at their highest.

But if you can get past the fifth day, you will likely see the cravings disappear, the clouds lift, and the body start to repair itself, releasing weight and giving you more energy.

I've noticed over the years that few people set out to accomplish their goals with a solid plan for how they will overcome obstacles along the way. This is especially true when you start a new diet or fitness regime: you tend to think only about how great you'll feel or look at the end of the program, failing to plan for the food cravings and temptations you'll likely encounter along the way. But if you plan for the obstacles, then you'll be prepared when they arise—and much more likely to overcome them and make it to your goal.

So as I walk you through the details of the 45-Day Reset in the third section of this book, I'll point out where I see patients hit these obstacles and what you can do to move through them as quickly and easily as possible.

Since you already know that the first five days will feel new and can be tough, you should create a support system around you that will cheer you on and remind you why you want to change. Write a letter to yourself telling you why this reset is so important to you. Read it on the night of Day 3. The important thing is to keep your eye on your *why*. And don't worry—in Part 3 of this book, I'll give you lots more ideas on how to stick with it. In fact, Chapter 8 is 100 percent focused on how to make sure you succeed with the 45-Day Reset!

What I love about this program more than anything is that it is built to wake up your inner doctor. Once that doctor gets a small taste that change is happening, it will go into massive repair mode. The more time you give the body to repair, the greater the result.

If weight loss is your prime objective, then the 45-Day Reset is perfect for you because it focuses on addressing the root of the weight problem. No more calorie counting, feeling hungry all the time, or isolating yourself to get the result you want.

As you reset your health, your metabolism is revved up. This will provide you with consistent and reliable energy that will have you burning fat without exercise. It's not about exercising for hours on end either. In fact, this program only requires short periods of exercise. What this program does is "reboot" your body. Its aim is to help your body go back to how it was before it started experiencing negative health symptoms. So get ready for your metabolism to be jumpstarted, your digestive system to be repaired, cravings to stop, and your body to function as it was designed to do.

I'm excited for you! The journey you are about to embark upon will have you feeling twenty again.

Part 2

How Your Body Functions— and Why It Breaks Down

CHAPTER 2

Your Gut Instincts Are Right

All disease begins in the gut.

—Hippocrates

ONE OF THE FIRST PLACES to go hunting for a breakdown in your health is in your gastrointestinal system. This system is also known as the GI tract, the digestive system, and the gut—which is what I like to call it. From this point forward, I will be referring to the entire gastrointestinal system as your *gut*, which includes all aspects of your digestion: your mouth, stomach, small intestine, and large intestine.

The gut has been called our second brain because so many other pieces of the body are controlled by this area. Immunity, key vitamins, neurotransmitters, and hormones are all affected by the health of your gut. Your gut is host to an incredible microbiome of bacteria that all have to be in balance in order for your brain and body to function at their best. If you want to reset your health, you need to reset your gut.

In this chapter, we'll talk about why the gut is so important to health, what the gut consists of, and what happens when different areas of the gut start to break down.

YOUR GUT: NUMBER ONE WHEN IT COMES TO HEALTH

Before I walk you through the typical breakdowns of the gut, I want you to understand some basic (and maybe even surprising!) functions that the gut performs. Most people know that this system is responsible for digesting food and converting it into nutrients that the body can use. But what many people don't know is that the gut has many other life-sustaining responsibilities as well.

To start with, your gut controls 70 to 80 percent of your immune system.[6] It's like a guard or a gatekeeper that signals the alarm to let your immune system know if there's an intruder like foreign bacteria, viruses, or fungi.

But your gut also manufactures critical elements required by the body for good health, including the following:

- ➢ Key vitamins (like the B's)
- ➢ Omega-3 amino acids. These are important for normal metabolism; they've been shown to reduce inflammation, improve cardiovascular health, and increase brain function.
- ➢ Serotonin, the "happy hormone." Serotonin helps with the regulation of mood, appetite, and sleep. It also supports cognitive functions such as memory and learning.

The gut also helps the body to absorb thyroid hormones like T3 and T4. These hormones are primarily responsible for regulation of metabolism; they're activated by the healthy bacteria of your gut.[7]

If your gut is not healthy, it's likely you'll have a catastrophic breakdown in your body. So how can you tell if your gut has been compromised?

---

6 J. B. Furness, Wolfgang A. Kunze, and Nadine Clerk, "Nutrient Tasting and Signaling Mechanisms in the Gut II: The Intestine as a Sensory Organ; Neural, Endocrine, and Immune Responses," *American Journal of Physiology* 277, no. 5, pt. 1 (1999): G922–28.

7 Andrew P. Halestrap and Marieangela C. Wilson, "The Monocarboxylate Transporter Family: Role and Regulation," *IUBMB Life* 64, no 2 (2012): 109–19.

If you have two or more of the following symptoms, there's a good chance your gut is out of balance and due for a reset:

- Trouble losing weight
- Depression, moodiness, anxiety, paranoia
- Bloating after you eat
- Chronic pain
- Fibromyalgia

- Fatigue
- Lack of focus
- Catching colds all the time
- Constipation
- Joint pain

THE GUT: WHAT IT LOOKS LIKE AND WHY IT BREAKS DOWN

To understand how easy it is for your gut to get out of balance, let's look at all the pieces that make up the gastrointestinal system and what lifestyle habits break those pieces down. As you look at each piece, you might see where your gut has gone astray. Make a note of it. Then, during your 15-Day Detox, we'll talk about how to put the health of your gut back on track again.

The gastrointestinal system comprises the mouth, the stomach, the small intestine, and the large intestine. Here's a closer look at each of these and what needs to happen to ensure that they work the way they're supposed to!

MOUTH

Believe it or not, digestion begins in your mouth. Chewing your food is massively important to digestion. When you chew your food, you release chemicals called enzymes that help you break down the food to prepare it for your stomach. What throws the gut off right from the start is (1) not chewing enough or (2) drinking with your meal.

Not chewing enough means that not enough enzymes are being released from your salivary glands. If food is not broken down enough in the mouth, you burden the stomach and ask it to do extra work. The same thing happens when you drink with your meals. You dilute those enzymes and reduce their effectiveness.

STOMACH

Most people think of their stomach as the main place that digestion happens. But really, the stomach's main purpose is temporary storage and the further breakdown of food. One way that the stomach does this is by secreting gastric acid, also known as HCL. HCL is important in preparing food for the small intestine. If you're low in HCL, foods such as proteins won't get broken down properly and will be sent in an undigested state to the small intestine, where they will ferment. This fermentation process creates an environment in which fungi like candida thrive. Candida is a huge health problem that we'll discuss in detail later in this chapter.

Signs That Your HCL Is Low

Your body will give you many signs when it's low in HCL. The following are key indications:

- Bloating, belching, and gas after a meal
- Indigestion, diarrhea, or chronic constipation
- Acne
- Rectal itching
- Chronic candida
- Hair loss in women
- Chronic fatigue
- Adrenal fatigue
- Various autoimmune diseases

Causes of Low HCL

The biggest culprits are these:

- High-carbohydrate sugary foods
- Medications
- Genetically modified foods
- Processed foods
- Chronic stress

SMALL INTESTINE

This is where the magic happens in the gut. If you can keep your small intestine healthy and happy, your whole body will perform at a higher level. Two key things must be kept in balance in your intestines: good bacteria and bad bacteria.

There are over one thousand different types of bacteria in the small intestine. As we noted earlier, we call these bacteria the microbiome of your body. In total, there are billions of bacteria in the small intestine—close to three-and-a-half pounds' worth! These bacteria are crucial to keeping your immune system functioning well, producing neurotransmitters, keeping B-vitamins and omega-3 levels high, activating your thyroid hormones, and ensuring that your serotonin levels are working at their best. You should have 80 percent good bacteria in your gut and 20 percent bad bacteria. If you get more than 20 percent bad bacteria from harmful foods you eat, you gut will be in trouble.

Small Intestinal Bacterial Dysbiosis (SIBO)

Small intestinal bacterial dysbiosis, or SIBO for short, is a complicated term for a condition in which a person's small intestine has too many of the bad bacteria and not enough of the good ones. When the intestines contain the balance of good and bad bacteria that is optimal for good health, the intestines are described as being in a state of symbiosis. Alternatively, *dysbiosis* (a contraction of the term "dys-symbiosis") occurs when this balance is upset. SIBO results when you have a deficiency in good bacteria and an overgrowth of bad bacteria.

Symptoms of SIBO include the following:

➤ Bloating, belching, burning, and flatulence after meals
➤ A sense of fullness after eating

➤ Indigestion, diarrhea, and constipation
➤ Systemic reactions after eating

- ➤ Nausea or diarrhea after taking supplements
- ➤ Rectal itching
- ➤ Weak or cracked fingernails
- ➤ Dilated capillaries in the cheeks and nose in nonalcoholic people
- ➤ Post-adolescent acne or other skin irritations, such as rosacea
- ➤ Iron deficiency
- ➤ Chronic intestinal infections, parasites, yeast, and unfriendly bacteria
- ➤ Undigested food in the stool
- ➤ Greasy stools
- ➤ Skin that's easily bruised
- ➤ Fatigue
- ➤ Amenorrhea (absence of menstruation)
- ➤ Chronic vaginitis (vaginal irritation)

As you might have noticed, some of these symptoms are similar to those resulting from low HCL production. That is how the digestive system works. Since digestion begins in the mouth and continues in the stomach, small intestine, and large intestine—all the way through the elimination process—if any piece of this digestive plan goes wrong, it will cause stress on the other pieces. One breakdown leads to another, until the whole system is in bad shape.

This is why a part of a 45-Day Reset includes a complete gut repair. You have to repair all the pieces to get the gut moving in the right direction and bring the body back into balance.

What causes SIBO? Here are some of the most common causes:

- ➤ Stress
- ➤ Diets that are poor or imbalanced and lacking nutritional supplementation; imbalanced diets may be extreme in carbohydrates, fat, or animal products
- ➤ Food allergies or sensitivities
- ➤ Frequent antibiotic or drug therapy
- ➤ Emotional stress
- ➤ Intestinal infections
- ➤ Parasite infestation
- ➤ Chronic inflammation

Candida

If you have an intense addiction to sugar, you need to pay close attention to what I have to say next. When you have more bad bacteria than good, you create an environment where yeast can grow. Foods that contain yeast—such as bread, beer, and sugary treats—ferment in your small intestine, building up a fungus called *candida*. Sounds gross, doesn't it?

Candida overgrowth can be one of the hardest gut situations to repair—mostly because this fungus needs you to consume more sugar, breads, starchy carbohydrates, and alcohol to keep it alive. It's like a parasite that tells you what to do so that you continue to build an environment that makes it happy. Candida is no joke.

Here are some telltale signs that you have candida:

➢ Skin and nail fungal infections (such as athlete's foot or toenail fungus)
➢ Feeling tired and worn down or suffering from chronic fatigue or fibromyalgia
➢ Digestive issues such as bloating, constipation, or diarrhea
➢ Autoimmune disease such as Hashimoto's thyroiditis, rheumatoid arthritis, ulcerative colitis, lupus, psoriasis, scleroderma, or multiple sclerosis (MS)
➢ Difficulty concentrating, poor memory, lack of focus, ADD, ADHD, and brain fog
➢ Skin issues, such as eczema, psoriasis, hives, and rashes
➢ Irritability, mood swings, anxiety, or depression
➢ Vaginal infections, urinary tract infections, rectal itching, or vaginal itching
➢ Severe seasonal allergies or itchy ears
➢ Strong sugar and refined carbohydrate cravings

I have personal experience with the devastation of candida. This was one of the major breakdowns in my body when I had Chronic Fatigue

Syndrome. Without even realizing it, I was a prime candidate for candida overgrowth. I had destroyed my gut bacteria by taking medications over the long term, and I was eating a diet high in breads, beer, and sugar.

One of the first steps to my healing was to kill candida—a process that can be brutal and can take time. Candida die-off can make you more fatigued and cause ringing in your ears, rashes, foggy brain, and achy joints. It took a thorough approach to kill candida in my body. It was tough, but boy, was it worth it!

Leaky Gut Syndrome

There's a new gut syndrome in town that's getting all the blame—and with good reason. It's called *leaky gut syndrome*. Leaky gut is being linked to a wide variety of symptoms, such as seasonal allergies, digestive problems, brain fog, hormonal imbalances, autoimmune disease, and chronic pain.

Leaky gut is a condition in which microholes form in your gut. These holes allow undigested food and toxins to enter into the bloodstream. The brain identifies these substances as foreign invaders and orchestrates an immune response. One of the body's greatest immune responses is inflammation. With leaky gut syndrome, it's as if someone turned on an inflammation switch. For some, leaky gut starts as inflammation in the belly, but for others, it creates inflammation in the back, neck, and extremities. The body's inflammatory repair system starts working 24/7, and your symptoms start getting worse and worse.

The following are signs that you might have leaky gut:

- ➢ Digestive issues such as gas, bloating, diarrhea, or irritable bowel
- ➢ Seasonal allergies or asthma
- ➢ Hormonal imbalances such as PMS or PCOS

- ➢ Diagnosis of an autoimmune disease such as rheumatoid arthritis, Hashimoto's thyroiditis, lupus, psoriasis, or celiac disease
- ➢ Diagnosis of chronic fatigue or fibromyalgia

➢ Mood and mind issues such as depression, anxiety, ADD, or ADHD

➢ Skin issues such as acne, rosacea, or eczema

➢ Diagnosis of candida overgrowth

➢ Food allergies or food intolerances

The worst part about leaky gut is that it wears down your body's immune system. An immune system that has been working on overdrive for years is ill equipped to fight diseases like cancer.

So what causes leaky gut? Gluten is the number one-cause (see the next section on food allergies). Other inflammatory foods—like dairy, processed foods, sugar, and alcohol—are suspected as well. Certain medications—like painkillers, antibiotics, and acid-reducing drugs—also lead to leaky gut. Candida overgrowth and SIBO are also known to contribute to this harmful gut situation.

Whenever I have a patient who has a variety of symptoms that don't seem to be resolving, I think of leaky gut. People who have had multiple surgeries or who have been taking medication for years to manage their symptoms seem to have the worst cases of leaky gut.

Large Intestine

Once the small intestine has pulled the nutrients from your food, it sends anything that can't be absorbed to your large intestine. The large intestine is responsible for breaking down the food even more by adding water to it.

One of the most important things to know about the large intestine is its connection to your skin. The health of your skin is a direct reflection of the health of your gut, especially the large intestine. Think of the large intestine as an excretion organ. It prepares any remaining undigested food for excretion—and one of the ways it excretes toxins is by pushing them out through the skin. Any toxins that irritate or destroy the lining of the large intestine will get sent into the bloodstream and out through the skin. Food allergies, especially allergies to dairy, destroy the large intestine.

WHY SO MANY FOOD ALLERGIES?

Have you noticed recently that everyone around you has a food allergy? Why is that? Well, unfortunately, we are not eating the same quality of food that we ate years ago. The following is a list of the top five food allergens and why they harm your gut.

WHEAT

Wheat is harmful to the human body for two reasons. The first is the new hybrid of wheat that we're eating. The second is what farmers are spraying on wheat crops today. In the 1970s, farmers discovered a smaller higher-yield dwarf version of wheat. This made for larger profits for the farmers but started an epidemic of digestive problems, autoimmune diseases, obesity, and behavioral challenges. Think back to when you were a kid—none of these conditions where prevalent at the rates they are now.

According to William Davis in his book *Wheat Belly*, this new hybrid of wheat is packed with several harmful proteins that destroy the lining of our guts and cross the blood-brain barrier, attaching themselves to the nervous system and opiate receptors in the brain. One of these proteins is called *gliadin*. When gliadin binds to opiate receptor sites in the brain, it induces appetite and causes behavioral changes. Such changes include outbursts, inattention in children with ADHD and autism, hearing voices, social detachment in schizophrenics, and mania in bipolar patients. Davis also states that people who take in gliadin consume four hundred more calories per day.

The second issue with wheat is what is allowed to be sprayed on it. Farmers are now spraying Roundup on wheat before they harvest it—yes, the same Roundup you use to kill weeds in your lawn. This spray has a chemical in it called *glyphosate*. Glyphosate causes microholes in our guts, causing leaky gut syndrome. Theses holes allow denatured pro-teins to cross through the gut lining into our blood, acting as foreign proteins. This stimulates our immune system and drives massive inflam-mation, more food allergies, and eventually disease.

Between the changes in wheat type and the spraying of toxic chemi-cals, can you see why so many people are allergic to wheat today? This is why you remove all wheat from your diet during your 45-Day Reset. I know this can be hard, but it's a necessary part of healing. If you don't give your gut a break from the daily damage this food substance is creat-ing, you will never heal. In fact, every day you stay committed to wheat, you risk building disease.

DAIRY

We weren't allergic to dairy as kids, were we? Now it seems as if everyone is allergic to dairy; in fact, it's estimated that 50 percent of the population is allergic. Well, just as with wheat, you're not consuming the same dairy as you did as a child. Milk, the primary ingredient in all dairy products, has been altered to increase production.[8] Just as the new version of wheat contains the harmful protein gliadin, milk has a new chain of amino ac-ids called BCM7—*beta a 1 casein*—better known as *casein*.

BCM7 produces reactions in your brain similar to those produced by morphine, and it can alter behavior and moods. If you have leaky gut, this protein goes right across the gut barrier and into your bloodstream, initiat-ing an immune response from your body. Your body reacts by inflaming to get this foreign invader out of you. Whether you're consuming conventional or organic dairy, you're getting this harmful protein. It's estimated that 95 percent of casein in America right now is this beta a1 version.

---

8 Gordana M. Kocic, Tatjana Jevtovic-Stoimenov, Dusan Sokolovic, and Hrstina Kocic, "Milk Consumption and Chronic Disease Risk: The Strategy or Challenge to Avoid and Eliminate 'Unwanted' Compounds and Contaminants," *Journal of Agricultural Science* 7, no. 5 (2015): http://www.ccsenet.org/journal/index.php/jas/article/view/45213/

Remember that I mentioned the benefits of enzymes that naturally occur in our body to help break down food? Well, dairy has a natural enzyme that helps the human body digest it. It's called *lactase*. When you pasteurize dairy, you destroy that enzyme, leaving the human gut ill equipped to handle the digestion of lactose in cow's milk. When dairy hits the gut undigested, it creates an immune response that has the body producing inflammation to break it down.

The other challenge we have with dairy is what's being done to cows to protect them from the unsanitary environments they're often living in. Growth hormone, antibiotics, and chemical-sprayed food all seep into the glass of milk you're drinking. Antibiotics are known to kill all good and bad bacteria in the gut, leading to intestinal dysbiosis, which we discussed earlier in this chapter.

If you don't have the right amount of good bacteria, your immune system will be depressed, your pain increased, and your moods altered—all from drinking milk. Every time you drink milk, you create an inflammatory reaction. If you have allergies, sinus issues, digestive issues, and skin challenges—or if you feel as if your immune system is depressed—take milk out of your diet for 30 days and see what happens.

CORN

You will find throughout this book that I reference foods made from genetically modified organisms (GMOs). If you're not familiar with GMO foods and what they're doing to your health, now is the time to educate yourself. GMO foods are engineered to have a toxin inside them called *BT toxin*. BT toxin causes an insect's stomach to explode, resulting in death. Of course our food industry is about increasing profits, not health. The presence of BT toxin in GMO crops is helpful to the farmer because he or she doesn't lose as many crops to insect damage.

Unfortunately, BT toxin has not been fully studied as to how it affects the human body. However, many believe this toxin is contributing to the growing number of cases of leaky gut syndrome. If we ingest BT toxin on a daily basis, then it does damage to us by creating microholes in our guts—just as it does damage to insects. What's even scarier is that some scientists believe that this toxin gets into our DNA and shares information with our bacteria, causing our bodies to begin to produce and secrete BT toxin, creating more intestinal dysbiosis even in the absence of GMO food.

Many countries have banned GMO foods because of the damaging effects they could have on our health. Unfortunately, GMO foods are not only legal but extremely prevalent in America. Food giants like Monsanto have also gone to great lengths to make sure there are no labeling laws to show us which products are GMO and which are non-GMO. This has created a catastrophic health crisis that people in America will be dealing with for years to come. But the good news is that one can get around GMO foods by always looking for the USDA organic symbol. Anything with the USDA organic stamp has passed the test for non-GMO foods.

Nevertheless, until better labeling laws are in place, I recommend you stay away from the foods that are most commonly genetically modified, like corn. Anything that is made from corn—corn oil, corn tortillas, corn flour, corn chips—has BT toxin in it. In the 45-Day Reset, I have you pull all corn out of your diet to give your gut a good reset from the damages GMO foods are causing.

SOY

Isn't soy a health food? That's what we were taught years ago. We know more now. And just like the other foods that are causing so many allergies, you are not eating the soy you ate years ago.

There are two challenges with soy. First, it produces a chemical called *phytoestrogen*, which mimics estrogen. Phytoestrogen is a plant sterol that can drive up estrogen in your system. Ingesting soy can create hormonal problems often seen with perimenopause and menopause. In fact, soy started to get more attention when breast cancer rates started to skyrocket. Breast cancer is often fueled by too much estrogen.

The other challenge we have with soy, and why it's under the food allergy section, is that it too is one of the most genetically modified crops. Eating it will not only stimulate more estrogen but will cause more BT toxin to enter your gut. Although eating USDA organic soy will eliminate the BT toxin issue, soy still produces too much estrogen in your body. There is no health benefit that outweighs the risk of this harmful food.

PEANUTS/EGGS

More than three million Americans now have some kind of nut allergy. The number of children with peanut allergies more than tripled between 1997 and 2008.[9] What is causing our children to be so allergic?

Although there is not one clear reason for all these allergies, there are many theories that might explain the increase in sensitivities to these foods. One theory as to why these foods are causing more allergies and histamine reactions is that these substances are mixed in some vaccines and flu shots as preservatives. We are vaccinating our children at higher rates than ever before: most children are getting 69 vaccine shots by the seventh grade. Along with the increase in vaccines, there has been an increase in allergies and asthma in children, as previously noted.

How could something meant to help a child cause damage? How would it create a food allergy? Think for a moment what the purpose of a vaccine is: to create an immune response. So when you get injected with a vaccine, your body recognizes everything in the vaccine as a foreign

---

9   Scott H. Sicherer, Anne Muñoz-Furlong, James H. Godbold, and Hugh A. Sampson, "US Prevalence of Self-Reported Peanut, Tree Nut, and Sesame Allergy: 11-Year Follow-Up," *Journal of Allergy and Clinical Immunology* 125, no. 6 (2010): 1322-326.

invader. The goal of the vaccine is to give you an immune response to the bacteria in the vaccine, but it doesn't just give an immune response to the bacteria—it can stimulate an immune response to everything in that vaccine. And according to the CDC, the following are preservatives that are put in vaccines:

- Aluminum
- Antibiotics
- Egg protein
- Formaldehyde
- Monosodium glutamate (MSG)

- Thimerosal (aka mercury)
- Soy
- Yeast

Why is egg used in a vaccine? Well, according to the CDC, vaccine viruses grow on eggs. These vaccine viruses are injected into fertilized hens' eggs and incubated for several days to allow the viruses to replicate. The virus-containing fluid is harvested from the egg and put into the vaccine. When the vaccine is injected into you, particles of egg still remain in the vaccine.

What about peanuts? In her book *The Peanut Allergy Epidemic*, Heather Fraser defines the connection between vaccines and peanut allergies. She explains that a class of vaccine ingredients called *excipients* is a likely suspect in the rapid increase in peanut allergies. Adding an excipient to a vaccine formula is necessary to help an injectable vaccine move into the bloodstream and to improve its effectiveness. In her book, Fraser well documents the addition of excipients that contain peanut oil and the rise in peanut allergies.

Let's think this through for a moment. If antibiotics, soy, and yeast are known destroyers of the microbiome of our guts, what happens when children get so many vaccines throughout their younger years? If the gut plays such a large role in the immune system, doesn't anything that damages the gut weaken the immune system? How many more toxins can our children take? If we are damaging our guts through foods, vaccines, and environmental toxins, what does this mean for the long-term health of our children?

Luckily, a few people are waking up to these truths. Although we have a long way to go with the number of toxins our children are exposed to, some doctors and scientists are starting to ask these difficult questions.

You will see many themes running throughout this book. One main theme is that toxins and foods we have altered are destroying our health. When I first learned about many of these toxins, I was overwhelmed. I even rejected some of the theories I had read. For example, the first time I read a book about cutting out all grains from your diet to improve your metabolism, I thought the author was crazy. I put the book down and didn't revisit it until I started hearing more and more people saying the same thing.

Although I was wheat-free at the time, I was not ready to give up my wheat-free treats containing other grains. Then one day, I got inspired to try a no-grain diet for myself. The results were almost immediate. First, I noticed my energy was high all day long. Normally, my energy would take a dip at 3:00 p.m. Once I gave up all grains, that dip went away. I also quickly dropped extra weight I was carrying at the time, never to regain it. I shocked myself. I was so happy with how my body felt and functioned that I never went back to grains as part of my regular diet again.

The choice is always yours. No one is putting a gun to your head and telling you to stop eating the foods that are harming your health. But as you read through the chapters of this book, if you find yourself rejecting some of the ideas, ask yourself what is worth more: the taste of a food or feeling fantastic?

I choose feeling fantastic any day!

MONICA'S STORY

Monica's story is a great example of how your whole health can break down from a breakdown in the gut. Monica came to me with extreme pain in her lower back. She had tried everything. Cortisone shots, powerful pain killers, yoga, massages, and sporadic chiropractic care had kept her from being disabled. But the pain was getting worse. It had become so bad that she couldn't bend over to put her pants or shoes on in the morning.

Knowing that I did corrective chiropractic and nutritional work, one of Monica's closest friends sent her to me. I immediately ran several tests on her and did a set of X-rays. The damage to her spine was severe. It would take several weeks for me to get her gut test results back, so we immediately started our corrective chiropractic protocol.

In the beginning, she noticed that her pain would diminish after the adjustments, only to return hours later. I gave her home exercises to loosen her ligaments, and that helped the pain levels as well. But something was still blocking her body from healing.

Then her gut tests results came back. She had one of the worst levels of bad bacteria I had ever seen in a patient.

We immediately put her on the 15-Day GI and Liver Detox—and the results were almost immediate. Within days her pain had declined by 50 percent. Her mobility started to come back and she could actually dress herself. She also had an unexpected result of quick weight loss. In 15 days she lost eight pounds, and her belly, which had felt bloated and distended for years, shrank.

The greatest part was that you could see the joy coming back to Monica's life. When you're in chronic pain and lose the function of your body, nothing in your life works right. Health is your greatest asset. Everything in your life requires that you live in a healthy body.

Monica is a great example of how key your gut is to many of the symptoms you may be experiencing. Leaky Gut, SIBO, and candida affect more than just the digestive tract. They affect your pain levels, your brain function, and your immune system. Repairing your gut can transform your life.

It did for Monica.

CHAPTER 3

Why the Brain Is Your Most Powerful Healing Tool

Anything that affects the gut will affect the brain.

—Dr. Charles Majors

THE BRAIN IS THE CONTROL center of the body. It controls the functioning of everything from the smallest cells to the most complex organs. Nothing happens in your body without communication from the brain—making it your most powerful healing tool. So a basic understanding of how the brain works is crucial to resetting your health for the long term.

I like to think of the brain as your best friend. You know that friend you can call on in your darkest hour? The one that will be there for you always? The friend that always wants to help and always has your back? That is your brain's relationship to your body. It constantly scans the body for cells that need to be repaired, systems that need to be coordinated, and tissue that needs more healing.

What most people don't realize is that *in order for your brain to function normally, you have to have a healthy gut.* The brain and the gut are so intimately connected that even neurologists are now linking depression, ADD, anxiety, and dementia to damage in the gut. Your brain also needs a good lymphatic system to detoxify itself. New studies are beginning to help us understand just how important the *dura mater,* the outer sheath around the brain and spinal cord, is in assisting in this detoxification.

Anything that harms the dura mater has the potential to slow down this detoxification process, leaving protein buildup in the brain—and damaging effects.

In this chapter, we'll look at how the microbial environment in your gut can have a dramatic effect on your moods. We'll also look at how the brain best detoxifies and what you can do to facilitate this necessary process.

Brain Health Starts in the Gut

The brain is composed of eighty-six billion neurons. Each neuron carries information, beginning in the *neural body*, then passing through a long thin cord called an *axon*, and then moving out through things called *dendrites*. Like traffic flowing on a highway, information gets sent as impulses across the axon and out through a dendrite, where it meets another dendrite of a neuron to carry the information onward.

The myelin sheath, which acts like a shield protecting a neuron, requires an ample amount of B vitamins to carry the messages across the axon with speed and accuracy. Ironically, B vitamins are produced in your gut. If your gut is out of balance and you're suffering from symptoms of leaky gut syndrome or intestinal dysbiosis, as we discussed in Chapter 2, you will not produce enough B vitamins or the proper amount of neurotransmitters. If you're low in these key nutrients, it affects your neural activity.

What that means to you is a lack of mental clarity, less focus, more forgetfulness, depression, and often chronic pain. Many of these symptoms are now being linked to low vitamin B and neurotransmitter levels due to a gut imbalance.

Fatigue and lack of focus are health crises that many people deal with on a daily basis. Many of my patients have tried to treat these symptoms medically, with little success. Feeling frustrated, they start blaming their poor health on aging or circumstances in their life. You may feel this way about your own health as well, but nothing could be further from the truth. Your brain was built to stay mentally sharp all day. It was designed to keep you happy, and your energy levels should stay constantly high throughout the day. Any change from that is not normal. It simply means there's a breakdown somewhere inside that needs to be addressed.

I'm often asked by corporations to speak to their employees about managing stress. One of my favorite questions to ask them is "Who wakes up energetic and stays that way all day?" No one raises their hand, and almost everyone laughs—as if I'm telling them a joke. What many people are unaware of is that fatigue, depression, and lack of mental clarity can arise from a breakdown in the gut. This is why I started with the gut in the last chapter: fix the gut and you help the brain function normally.

When I started my practice twenty years ago, digestive problems were rare, as was depression. Now when I meet with a new patient and run through his or her health history, it's rare for someone to say they *don't* have some type of digestive challenge. The same is true with depression. I'm also seeing more and more people on antidepressants.

In fact, digestive complaints are so common now that a new survey conducted at New York University's Langone Medical Center found that 74 percent of Americans are living with digestive symptoms such as diarrhea, gas, bloating, and abdominal pain.[10] Anxiety and depression are also on the rise. According to the CDC, 1 out of 10 Americans over the age of 12 is now taking an antidepressant. That is a 400 percent increase since 1988.

It's not a coincidence that depression and anxiety are rising at similar rates. There's a connection. A growing amount of research is proving that an imbalance in the digestive system can cause imbalances in the

---

10 "Survey Shows 74 Percent of Americans Living with GI Discomfort," *Fox News Health*, November 24 2013, http://www.foxnews.com/health/2013/11/22/survey-shows-74-percent-americans-experience-gi-discomfort/

brain, leading to depression and changes in mood. In his book *Brain Maker*, David Perlmutter, MD, a board-certified neurologist, claims there is a medical revolution underway that has brain experts looking and treating behavioral and mood disorders, Alzheimer's disease, depression, ADD, dementia, and multiple sclerosis in a whole new way. According to Dr. Perlmutter, the health of your brain is dictated by the state of the *microbiome* in your gut—the ecosystem that houses all your body's microbes.

Mark Hyman, MD, asserts in his book *The UltraMind Solution,* "Your entire body and all of the core systems in it interact as a single sophisticated symphony. You are one whole person, and all the pieces of your biology and your unique genetic code interact with your environment (including the foods you eat) to determine how sick or well you are in this moment."[11]

For the first time in recent medical history, doctors are looking for answers to people's mental conditions in the gut. Traditionally, mental disorders have been treated with medication. SSRIs are drugs that are commonly given to patients with depression. But what is the purpose of an SSRI? It's to increase the serotonin levels in your body. What does serotonin do? It makes you happy. Where is this amazing chemical made? You guessed it: your gut.

Serotonin is a neurotransmitter. Neurotransmitters are essential for electrical impulses to be sent from neuron to neuron. This is how our thoughts occur. As noted earlier, information speeds along a neuron to the axon; it's with the help of a neurotransmitter that a neuron can connect to the next neuron and keep carrying the information along. *And neurotransmitters are made in the gut.* If your gut is out of balance, not secreting enough of the proper neurotransmitter, it will negatively affect how your brain functions.

---

11   Mark Hyman, *The UltraMind Solution: Fix Your Broken Brain by Healing Your Body First; The Simple Way to Defeat Depression, Overcome Anxiety, and Sharpen Your Mind* (New York: Scribner, 2008).

Remember how I said your brain is your best friend? Imagine if your best friend were down, not feeling well, depressed, or depleted of energy. How well would he or she be able to help you in a crisis? Not very well, I imagine. That same thing happens to your brain when it doesn't get the proper balance of neurotransmitters.

A deficiency in neurotransmitters can cause a wide variety of health problems:

➢ Sleep difficulties, including problems falling asleep, waking frequently in the middle of the night, and not being able to fall asleep after waking at night

➢ Craving refined carbohydrates

➢ Having a hard time dealing with life changes

➢ Difficulty relaxing; tension

➢ Low libido; lack of interest in sex

➢ Fatigue, even during the morning

➢ Lack of concentration

➢ Difficulty losing weight

➢ Eating too much sugar

➢ Depression

➢ Feeling taken advantage of by others

➢ Chronic fatigue

➢ Chronic pain

➢ Emotional volatility; mood swings you feel you can't control

➢ Difficulties in your family and work relationships because of moodiness

➢ Depression and feelings of isolation

➢ Excessive perspiration, cold hands, and palpitations

➢ Memory difficulties

➢ Difficulty overcoming even minor obstacles to achieve goals

➢ A tendency to dwell on your inadequacies and feel depressed

Do you see any of these symptoms in yourself?

One of the tests I often run in my office is an Organic Acids Test. It's a functional medicine test that helps me see if a person is low in B vitamins and neurotransmitters. It also tells me how depleted a patient's liver is of essential nutrients like glutathione, how much bad bacteria and yeast they have in their gut, and how quickly their cells are living and dying due to free-radical damage. It is a powerful test. I can see how quickly the person is building disease and identify some of the breakdowns that are contributing to the patient's poor health.

Recently I ran this test on a 40-year-old woman who had a long history of depression. She had had her depression under control for several years, but recently it had started to come back. This time the medication she was taking wasn't helping. She was teary often. She couldn't see the bright side of life, and it was starting to really impact her family. She was scared and frustrated.

When I ran the Organic Acids Test on her, sure enough, her body was packed with bad bacteria and low in neurotransmitters—a combination I often find. A simple fix of a high-powered probiotic and amino acids corrected the problem. Her story is such a good reminder to always ask why a new condition has arisen with your health. Don't just treat the symptom, treat the why (the breakdown). This approach to people's health has never steered me wrong. This woman, for example, most definitely would have ended up on higher-powered medications that would have caused more damage to her gut, making her neurotransmitter imbalance even worse.

Unfamiliar with neurotransmitters? Have you heard of GABA? It's a neurotransmitter that mellows you out and slows your thoughts down. Pretty helpful when you have a high-stress life, don't you think? Norepinephrine and epinephrine are also neurotransmitters that make you alert and give you that shot of adrenaline when you need it. And dopamine is the neurotransmitter that keeps your spirits high. These neurotransmitters are all crucial to happy living, and they are all made in the gut and sent to the brain. Keeping the microbiome of your gut well balanced will keep your brain loaded with these powerful chemicals.

Advances in neuroscience are showing us another interesting function of neurotransmitters: they have a profound impact on our habits. They glue patterns of thoughts together. When you think a thought over and over again, the neurotransmitters that get released at that time will hard-wire you to keep thinking that thought.[12] Let's use going on a diet as an example. One of the reasons that so many people fail at diets is that they have negative associations with the word *diet*. Most people have been on diets over and over again. Many have failed. The more times you fail at a diet, the more you hardwire your brain to associate the word *diet* with suffering and failure. All someone has to do is say the word "diet," and you feel horrible. Once this is hardwired through your neurons with the help of the neurotransmitters, it's hard to change. You're already programmed to fail.

But neuroscience has taught us some new information about this gluing of neurons together. Just like thoughts that get thought over and over again become hardwired in our brain, if you change a habitual thought to a new and better thought, you can unstick the neurons associated with that thought and eventually change the thought itself. You literally can undo your thoughts (and reset your brain).

You can use this to your advantage. When you get to the section on the 45-Day Reset, you are never going to call it a diet. If someone asks you what you're doing, you'll say, "I'm on a reset program," or "I'm resetting my health." Your association with the word *program* is totally different from that with the word *diet*. In fact, I want to emphasize that the 45-Day Reset is *not* a diet. It is a way of life. It is a toolset that will change the way you approach your health—and your health will change as a result.

THE CENTRAL NERVOUS SYSTEM

Now that you have a general understanding of the brain and how it plays a part in your health, let's look at the rest of your central nervous system. The nervous system is the brain's only messenger system. It carries information from the brain to every cell, tissue, muscle, and organ in your body. There are only two key concepts to know about this system.

---

12 R. Douglas Fields, "Beyond the Neuron Doctrine," *Scientific American Mind* 17, no.=
3 (2006): 20–27.

First, we have two types of nervous systems, designed to work in balance: one that speeds us up and one that slows us down. The one that speeds us up is called our *sympathetic* nervous system. The one that slows us down is called our *parasympathetic* nervous system. Most people are overusing their sympathetic nervous system. Our crazy-busy lifestyle has us on the go all the time. We are constantly running from event to event, causing us to constantly use our sympathetic nervous system.

Since the two systems were designed to work in balance, if you're constantly on the go, you most likely have overdeveloped your sympathetic nervous system, thus weakening your parasympathetic nervous system. An imbalance in these two systems can dramatically affect how well your body performs—and it can be the fast path to chronic fatigue.

So how would you know if one or both of these systems were out of balance? Following are some possible symptoms:

➢ Your brain races, especially at night.
➢ You find it hard to relax, even when you're exhausted.
➢ You never let you brain relax. In fact, it's difficult for you to just sit.
➢ You're addicted to your smartphone, checking e-mail and social media constantly.

Think of your two nervous systems like the gas pedal and brake of your car. If all you did was use the gas pedal and never the brake, you would eventually crash. What I want to do is teach you how to use the brake.

There are ways for you to develop your parasympathetic nervous system. Meditation is one way. Sitting for as little as ten minutes a day can strengthen your parasympathetic nervous system. I also recommend a technique called 4-7-8 breathing: inhale through your nose for a count of 4, hold the breath for a count of 7, and exhale from your mouth for a count of 8. If you do this several times, you will feel your body relaxing. It's quick, easy, and a wonderful way to strengthen your parasympathetic nervous system.

The second thing you need to know about the nervous system is that it is of such importance to your health and well-being that it has a bony case, called your spine, protecting it. Anything that damages your spine will damage your nervous system. If you damage your nervous system, you greatly impact your brain's ability to communicate with your body. This weakening of the nervous system can lead to many symptoms, including the following:

- Digestive problems
- Asthma
- Allergies
- Sinus problems
- Headaches

- Neck pain
- Lower back pain
- Lack of mental clarity
- Sluggish metabolism
- Infertility

Our spine was designed to have curves. The spinal cord that carries life-sustaining information out of the brain is designed to be seventeen to eighteen inches long, and the curvature of the spine helps maintain the length of the spinal cord. When we lose those curves, we pull and pinch the spinal cord and nerves. This greatly affects how well our brain can coordinate the functioning of all the cells of the body. Unfortunately, our sedentary lifestyle and technology is quickly damaging the curves in our spine.

What this means is that posture is not just about looking good. Posture tells you a lot about the health of your spine and whether these curves are still intact. In Chapter 7, I'll show you how to bring some of those curves back and restore the function of your nervous system with ease.

THE BRAIN'S LYMPHATIC SYSTEM

As I mentioned in the first part of this chapter, your brain also has a lymphatic system. When this system is functioning properly, it helps remove protein buildup and toxins believed to be related to neurodegenerative diseases such as ALS, Alzheimer's, and Parkinson's.

A recent study published in the *Journal of Neuroscience* shows that body posture has a profound effect on the efficiency of the brain's lymphatic system. More evidence shows that posture plays a key role in your overall health. Also, current research is showing us that sleep has an effect on how well this lymphatic system works. Getting enough sleep and sleeping on your side is said to help improve lymphatic drainage from the brain and help with memory consolidation. This drainage is key to preventing the neurodegenerative diseases mentioned above, such as Alzheimer's, Parkinson's, and ALS.

Yet one poor health habit I often hear about from patients is not getting enough sleep. The National Sleep Foundation says that most adults need seven to nine hours of sleep to function properly. Sleep is so important to your overall health that missing out on it will weaken your body. The Mayo Clinic states that studies are showing that people who don't get enough sleep are more likely to get sick after being exposed to a virus. Lack of sleep can also affect how fast you recover if you do get sick. When you're asleep, your brain can do its best work. Lack of sleep prevents this powerful healing tool from doing its job effectively.

It's important to know several things about sleep. First, the amount of sleep you get is important. In order for your brain to be able to repair itself properly, you need seven to nine hours of sleep each night. Not getting enough sleep has been found to do the following:

- Decrease the cognitive function of your brain
- Increase your risk of heart disease, heart attacks, strokes, and diabetes
- Kill your sex drive
- Lead to depression

- Age your skin
- Make you forgetful
- Make you gain weight by increasing the hormone that makes you hungry
- Increase your risk of death

When you go to sleep is also important. When the sun goes down, your body secretes melatonin to make you sleepy and to tell you to go to bed so it can start to repair injured cells. Four hours after the sun goes down, you should be in a deep REM sleep. This is usually pretty easy for people in the summertime. In the winter, however, it gets dark earlier. If you follow the above theory, you would have to go to bed by nine o'clock. This is difficult for many and might explain why more people get sick in the winter than in the summer. I like to use the general rule of getting seven to nine hours' sleep, so you should be in a deep sleep by 11:00 p.m. since most of the repair of your body happens between 11:00 p.m. and 2:00 a.m.

NOURISHMENT FOR THE BRAIN

I have great news for you: one of the key nutrients that your brain needs to function properly is good fat. Yes, you heard me right: fat nourishes the brain.

One growing concern that doctors are having with patients with Alzheimer's and dementia is that when a person is put on statin drugs for decades, it shuts down the liver's ability to produce cholesterol. Your brain needs some cholesterol to function normally. When the brain is void of good fat combined with an increase in toxins, a bad situation is created. Presently, one out three seniors will die with dementia or Alzheimer's. And what have we done over the past several decades? Removed fat from our diets and added in toxins. Could it be that these two, combined, are contributing to mental decline in our seniors?

So what kinds of fat does your brain need? Omega-3 fish oils are some of the best fats to add into your diet to nourish your brain. One of the largest studies (of twenty-two thousand people) ever done on the effects of omega-3's revealed that those who regularly took cod liver oil, which is rich in omega-3 fatty acids, were about 30 percent less likely to have symptoms of depression than those who did not. The study also showed that the longer the participants took cod liver oil, the less likely they were to have high levels of depression.

According to Douglas London, MD, Research Associate in Psychiatry at Harvard Medical School, "The human brain is 60 percent fat, and omega-3 fatty acids are the fatty acid of choice for the structure of certain parts of brain cell membranes and brain intercellular nerve connections. Lack of dietary omega-3 forces the brain cells to utilize other fatty acid on hand, resulting in cells constructed with inferior building material. This lack of available omega-3's affects brain function and is associated with cognitive and emotional disorders. There is growing evidence that a significant proportion of the US population is at risk for omega-3 fatty acid deficiency."[13]

This is why you'll see a fairly large dose of omega-3 fish oils included in your 45-Day Reset. You also will be adding in plenty of wild salmon, flaxseed oil, Brussels sprouts, and raw walnuts into your diet, as they are very high in omega-3's.

FINDING THE CAUSE TO REBALANCE THE BODY

Are you starting to understand how complex your body can be? All systems are interconnected, and this is why treating symptoms is a dead-end road that will never lead to restoring health. If you're having chronic fatigue because of a B-vitamin and neurotransmitter deficiency, and if you take a pill to try to fix it, then all you'll do is block your brain's ability to be aware of the fatigue. You won't have addressed the B-vitamin and neurotransmitter deficiency.

Your body wants to be in a state of balance and health. Symptoms are your body's way of letting you know that it's out of balance and needs assistance in restoring its health. So when you take a pill to mask your symptoms, your body will often develop another symptom to get your attention. This is why so often people get on one medication that throws their body even further out of balance, thus requiring another medication to take care of that new symptom.

---

13 Quoted in Laurie Barclay, "Report: Fighting Depression and Improving Cognition with Omega-3 Fatty Acids," *Life Extension Magazine*, October 2007, http://www.lifeextension.com/magazine/2007/10/report_depression/Page-01?p=1/

David's Story

Attention deficit hyperactivity disorder (ADHD) is a challenge that many parents are having to face every day with their children. Many parents are looking for solutions other than putting their child on lifelong medications with harmful side effects.

David's family was in this exact place when they came to see me. David was a second grader who was full of life, exuberant, curious—and incredibly unfocused. This made it difficult for his teachers to work with him in a classroom setting. His outbursts were often disruptive to the learning environment of the classroom. David's teachers recommended that the family seek outside help for his ADHD.

Numerous experts agreed that David should be put on medication, but David's mom refused to believe that was her only option. She started looking into how foods affected the attention of a young child. She pulled all processed foods, sugar, and toxins out of his food and their household. David's attention improved, but he was still a difficult child to have in the classroom. Continuing to search for answers, David's mom found my office. I X-rayed David and found that his top cervical vertebra was grossly misaligned. No doubt it was impacting how his brain was functioning and communicating with his body.

I started a protocol of care to realign David's atlas and strengthen the surrounding tissues. Within a month, changes started to happen. It started with David's teacher commenting that he could sit for longer periods of time.

Then she showed David's mother handwriting samples: his letters were more clear and well formed. Another month went by and David was an all but normal child in the classroom—still his spunky self but much more focused and able to participate in classroom activities in a respectable way.

David's story is a perfect example of how we treat the symptom and not the cause. Once we took pressure off his brainstem, his whole body relaxed and his brain could function the way it was designed to.

CHAPTER 4

Reward Your Hardest Working Organ—Your Liver

*The food that you eat can either be the safest and most
powerful medicine or the slowest form of poison.*

—Ann Wigmore

THE LIVER IS THE HARDEST working organ in the body. The small intestine filters the toxins we ingest and sends them to the liver to break them down to facilitate their exit from the body. So the liver performs functions related to the digestive process, metabolism, immunity, and hormonal control. It also plays a role in cleaning up the body: getting rid of toxins and waste, as well as drugs and other foreign chemicals. The liver is a ridiculously important organ—which is why one of the keys to resetting your health is resetting this organ.

Although gaining a complete understanding of how the liver works can be a daunting task, learning a few key concepts about it will help you take care of this amazing organ. In this chapter, we'll look at how the liver works, what foods and substances harm the liver, and why resetting the liver is one of the very first things we do in the 45-Day Reset.

THE MIRACULOUS LIVER

The cells of the liver screen and filter the blood. The liver is so well built that it actually has specialized cells specifically designed to metabolize drugs and alcohol. Any toxic substances are deactivated and rearranged for eventual excretion.

Because detoxification is its specialty, the liver also produces a substance called *glutathione*. Production of glutathione is one of those things your body was designed to do naturally. Glutathione helps recycle and extend the life of your body's important antioxidants. It also helps to directly remove toxins from your various systems. It acts like a magnet, binding toxins and free radicals and rendering them inactive and easy to excrete. Once these toxins and free radicals are bound, they can be incorporated into the bile and brought to the digestive tract to be excreted via the stool. Free radicals are a killer of health and speed up the aging process, so getting them out of your body is extremely beneficial.

The problem—and it's a major problem most people are facing today—is that our glutathione levels are being depleted by harmful toxins and other factors we encounter on a daily basis. The key things that deplete our glutathione levels are medications, aging, stress, pollution, radiation exposure, and poor diet. They can decrease the liver's capability to detoxify the blood, causing toxin buildup and increased oxidative stress. This in turn can increase a person's risk of diseases, such as cancer, diabetes, and heart disease—and it can accelerate the aging process.

You will hear me say this over and over: the environment we're living in is more toxic than ever. Our liver has a tougher job than it did decades ago. Being mindful of what foods are hardest on the liver and incorporating a good detox several times a year is crucial for the health of your digestion, metabolism, and immune system.

TOXINS THAT DEPLETE YOUR GLUTATHIONE LEVELS

Following is a list of toxins and other factors that can deplete your natural glutathione levels:

- Acetaminophen (Tylenol) and other pharmaceuticals
- Acetone, solvents, and paint removers
- Fuels and fuel by-products

- Heavy metals (mercury in dental amalgams, vaccines, and tattoos; lead; cadmium; and copper)
- Pesticides and herbicides

- Nitrates and other food preservatives of chemical origin (in salami, hot dogs, hams, bologna, smoked foods, etc.)
- Artificial sweeteners, like Aspartame
- Synthetic food dyes
- Benzopyrenes (tobacco smoke, barbequed foods, fuel exhaust, etc.)
- Alcohol
- Household chemicals (synthetically scented and colored detergents and fabric softeners, air fresheners, mothballs, mildew removers, cleaners and bleach, lawn and plant fertilizers, etc.)
- Chemicals found in housewares (nonstick coating used in pans and skillets, plastic containers and linings of tin cans and other food packaging)
- Formaldehyde (in vaccines and flu shots)
- Styrene (found in photocopiers and toner printers)

- Chlorine in treated water
- Medical X-rays
- UV radiation
- Electromagnetic fields (EMFs) (like the ones coming from your cell phone, tablets, and laptops)
- Industrial pollutants
- Poor diet (see 45-Day Reset)
- Strenuous exercise (This is why we recommend Surge Training.)
- Chronic stress
- Anxiety and depression (Fixing the gut will help this.)
- Light pollution (Bed lights, streets lights, and the blue light from phones and tablets all suppress melatonin production at night. Melatonin is key for glutathione production.)
- Age (After the age of 20, natural glutathione production decreases at the rate of 10 percent per decade on average in healthy adults.)

Many of you may be looking at this list and thinking *I'm exposed to many of those toxins. How is this affecting my health? What can I do about it?* This is one of the main reasons I've written this book. We're exposed to so many things on a daily basis that are destroying our health, and many of us are completely unaware of this. People are walking around fearful of cancer, yet they don't realize that their daily habits are building cancer within them every day. In fact, a top British medical journal, the *Lancet*, found that glutathione levels were highest in healthy young people, lower in healthy elderly people, even lower in sick elderly people, and the lowest of all in hospitalized elderly people.[14] Bottom line: if you're sick and need a reset, you have to get these glutathione levels up.

The first step to fixing anything is knowing that it's broken. Just knowing that these toxins are depleting your glutathione levels, thus accelerating the disease and aging process, is the first step. The second step is minimizing your exposure to these toxins. The third step is finding ways to detoxify your liver and improve your glutathione levels. The 15-Day GI and Liver Detox will help with this third step, as will following very specific steps you can take to improve your glutathione levels.

WAYS TO IMPROVE YOUR GLUTATHIONE LEVELS
Just as your habitual daily activities deplete your glutathione levels, you can add in daily activities that improve your levels. These habits include the following:

CONSUME SULFUR-RICH FOODS
The main sulfur-rich foods in the diet are garlic, onions, and cruciferous vegetables (broccoli, kale, cabbage, cauliflower, watercress, etc.)

TRY BIOACTIVE WHEY PROTEIN
This is a great source of cysteine and the amino acid building blocks for glutathione synthesis. The trick with whey protein is that it has to be a

---

14   S. L. Nuttall, U. Martin, A. J. Sinclair, and M. J. Kendall, "Glutathione: In Sickness and in Health," *The Lancet* 351, no. 9103 (1998): 645–46.

very specific type: it MUST be bioactive and made from non-denatured proteins (*denaturing* refers to the breakdown of the normal protein structure). When choosing whey protein, make sure it is derived from non-pasteurized and non-industrially produced milk from grass-fed cows. It's also important that the ingredients say there are no pesticides, hormones, or antibiotics.

Whey protein is found in protein powders. There are thousands of protein powders on the market, and it's easy to be misled by a bad product. Please go to Resetfactor.com to see my preferred brands, which meet the criteria mentioned above.

EXERCISE BOOSTS YOUR GLUTATHIONE LEVELS

If you need more reasons to exercise, here's a great one: exercise increases your glutathione levels, thus boosting your immune system, improving your body's ability to detox, and enhancing your body's antioxidant defenses. The best type of exercise to increase these levels is Surge Training (mentioned in the 45-Day Reset chapter). Surge Training is an exercise technique in which you work to get your heart rate up and down over a 15-minute time period. It's quick and effective.

Strength training is another powerful way to improve your glutathione levels. We have become a treadmill culture, where we hop on a treadmill going at the same pace for a long period of time. In Chapter 5, "Calories Don't Count—Hormones Do," you'll see how ineffective I believe this type of exercise to be. Surge and strength training for short periods are the most beneficial way to improve your glutathione levels and get in amazing shape.

TAKE GLUTATHIONE-SUPPORTING SUPPLEMENTS

Some people ask, "If glutathione is so crucial to my overall health, can't I just take a pill for it?" Well, the answer is no. The challenge with glutathione is that it's a protein. When you ingest proteins, the body will break them down by digesting them and you won't get the amazing benefits that glutathione offers. But the great thing is that the production of glutathione in the body requires many different nutrients that you CAN take. The following are key ingredients your body can use to produce more glutathione:

1. **N-acetyl-cysteine.** This has been used for years to help treat asthma and lung disease and to treat people with life-threatening liver failure caused by excessive Tylenol use.
2. **Alpha lipoic acid.** This is a close second to glutathione in importance for our cells. It is involved in energy production, blood sugar control, brain health, and detoxification. The body usually makes it, but given all the stress we're under, we are often depleted in this key nutrient.
3. **Methylation nutrients** (folate and vitamins B6 and B12). These are perhaps the most critical to keeping the body producing glutathione. Methylation and the production and recycling of glutathione are the two most important biochemical functions in your body. Take folate, B6, and B12.
4. **Selenium.** This important mineral helps the body recycle and produce more glutathione.
5. **Vitamins C & E.** These two vitamins work together to recycle glutathione.
6. **Milk thistle (silymarin).** This has long been used in liver disease and to boost glutathione levels.

You'll notice in the 45-Day Reset chapter that I recommend these key supplements to stimulate your glutathione levels. As with all the supplements I recommend in this book, you can go to Resetfactor.com to see my favorite ones and where you can order them from. Choosing supplements can be confusing. Don't let overwhelming amounts of information or lack of clarity keep you from getting these key nutrients. I want you to get results.

OTHER FOODS TOXIC TO THE LIVER

Many of the foods we're eating are harming our liver. Here are some foods known to destroy your liver quickly:

FAST FOOD

No surprise here, right? A study from Europe showed that eating too much fast food—resulting in a diet that's high in fat and sugar (including high-fructose corn syrup)—could cause serious damage to the liver. Follow-up studies also showed, however, that such damage could be reversed by giving up the unhealthy diet.

According to Dr. Andrew Ordon, author of *Better in 7*, a new study has found that eating fast food for a month can cause significant changes to your liver.[15] The combination of bad fats, sugar, and salt causes something called fatty liver disease. Fatty liver disease can be found in both obese and thin people. The United States has 160,000 fast food restaurants serving an estimated fifty million customers every day. Dr. Ordon states that the changes you can see in liver enzymes after one month of eating french fries are in line with the effects doctors see with hepatitis.

Think about that. Fifty million people every day are damaging their liver just by eating fast food. This harmful daily habit—along with other harmful habits such as sedentary living, consuming a diet that causes a lack of good bacteria in the gut, and engaging in behaviors that damage the nervous system—is destroying people's health. Can you begin to see why more and more people are getting cancer? Is it starting to make

---

15 "Fried Foods Have Similar Impact on Your Liver as Hepatitis," *CBS News,* February 16, 2013, http://www.cbsnews.com/news/fried-foods-have-similar-impact-on-your-liver-as-hepatitis/

sense why we live in one of the sickest countries in the industrial world? Can you see why people desperately need to be educated and given tools to reset their health?

ALCOHOL

Another no-brainer. Too much alcohol can lead to liver disease. Alcohol turns healthy liver cells into fat. Because the liver has no cells that can feel these changes, most people that drink on a regular basis don't realize they're damaging their liver until it's too late.

When you drink a glass of alcohol, it is so stressful to the liver that the liver can only focus on one thing at that moment: metabolizing that alcohol. As long as that alcohol is in your system, you are not burning fat or detoxifying. The average glass of alcohol takes ten hours for the liver to process. This is why I have you take alcohol out during your 45-Day Reset.

The other aspect of alcohol that's important to understand is the fact that many alcoholic beverages have yeast in them. As I mentioned in the gut chapter, yeast is a bad fungus that will destroy your gut. The more yeast you have, the sicker your gut will be. Drinking alcohol irritates the lining of the stomach, gradually weakening the kidneys and liver and leading to serious health problems. Remember that anything that destroys the gut and liver interferes with healthy metabolism and the weight loss process.

SALT

There are so many misconceptions about salt—it's really gotten a bad rap. But very much like fats, there are good salts and bad salts. Table salt is bad salt. It is highly processed and stripped of key minerals your body needs. You know that too much table salt can increase blood pressure, but did you know that it can also lead to fatty liver disease?

Here's why. Table salt is not just sodium chloride. It contains additives that are designed to make it more free-flowing: ferrocynanide, talc, and silica aluminate are commonly included. Aluminum accumulates inside the body and can harm the nervous system, even leading to neurological disorders. Talc is a known carcinogen. How can companies that produce table salt put a known carcinogen in foods we eat every day? Well, the FDA has a special provision allowing talc in table salt, even while it is prohibited in all other foods due to toxicity issues. According to current regulations, table salt can be up to 2 percent talc.

What's the best alternative to table salt? Sea salt. Unlike table salt, sea salt is unrefined and unadulterated, and it's not harmful in moderate amounts. Its benefits are vast. The human body requires a certain amount of sodium for optimum health; we can't live without some sodium. Healthy sea salts make your body a hostile environment for pathogens such as bad bacteria and parasites. This is what makes sea salt such an excellent preservative.

Sea salt also contains selenium, which helps to chelate toxic metals from the body. This is extremely helpful to the liver. Sea salt also contains boron, which helps prevent osteoporosis; and chromium, which regulates blood sugar levels. Sea salt is one of the few sources of copper that is safe to ingest, and copper helps the body to form new arteries whenever the main arteries become too clogged. Consuming small quantities of sea salt will actually lower your blood pressure.[16]

Adding sea salt to your daily health regime will also help with your metabolism. Mineral deficiencies are partly responsible for the rising obesity epidemic. Obese people are often malnourished, and ironically their bodies are starving for key minerals and nutrients. When your body thinks it's starving, it will hold on to fat, only intensifying the obesity challenge that many people face. So can you see that it's time to throw away the table salt and add in the sea salt! Both your liver and your metabolism will thank you.

---

16 Melinda Wenner Moyer, "It's Time to End the War on Salt," *Scientific American*, July 8, 2011, http://www.scientificamerican.com/article/its-time-to-end-the-war-on-salt/

ARTIFICIAL SWEETENERS

Next to alcohol, some of the worst foods you can eat or drink contain aspartame or sucralose—which go under the brand names Splenda, NutraSweet, and Equal. These foods will NEVER make you thinner and will destroy your health every time. They are so harmful that our government has advised that pregnant women and children should avoid them.

Aspartame accounts for over 75 percent of the adverse reactions to food additives reported to the FDA.[17] Many of these reactions are very serious, including seizures and death. Over 90 different documented symptoms have been reported as part of the dangers of aspartame. These symptoms include the following:

- Headaches
- Dizziness
- Seizures
- Nausea
- Numbness
- Muscle spasms
- Weight gain
- Rashes
- Depression
- Fatigue
- Irritability
- Tachycardia and heart palpitations

- Insomnia
- Vision problems
- Hearing loss
- Breathing difficulties
- Anxiety attacks
- Memory loss
- Tinnitus
- Vertigo
- Joint pain
- Loss of taste

There is no doubt that aspartame is one of the most harmful food substances you can put in your mouth. According to researchers and physicians studying the adverse effects of aspartame, several severe illnesses can be triggered or worsened by ingesting aspartame. These include the following:

---

17 "Aspartame: By Far the Most Dangerous Substance Added to Foods Today," Mercola website, November 6, 2011, http://articles.mercola.com/sites/articles/archive/2011/11/06/aspartame-most-dangerous-substance-added-to-food.aspx.

- Brain tumors
- Multiple Sclerosis
- Epilepsy
- Chronic Fatigue Syndrome
- Parkinson's disease

- Alzheimer's disease
- Lymphoma
- Fibromyalgia
- Diabetes

If you're still not convinced that now is the time to get off this harmful chemical, current studies done on rats show that aspartame increases the incidence several types of cancer, especially liver and lung cancer.[18] Because of the numerous harmful effects of aspartame and the growing awareness of these effects, more people have started to switch to sucralose, better known as Splenda. Sucralose is not proving to be any safer. One study showed that mice had a higher risk of developing cancer after eating sucralose. Other side effects reported with Splenda include the following:

- Rashes
- Dizziness
- Migraines
- Stomach pain

- Diarrhea
- Bladder irritation
- Numbness

You will find aspartame and sucralose in many low-fat or nonfat foods. This is why one of my reset rules for health is that you have to start reading labels. Read your labels and stay away from these harmful ingredients at all cost.

Aspartame was one of the toxins that led me to chronic fatigue syndrome. Back in college, it would not have been uncommon for me to have three super gulp–sized diet Cokes every day. Between the chronic daily painkillers I was taking, the stress I was under, the diet Cokes, and the fast food, I was a prime candidate for chronic fatigue syndrome and didn't know it. My liver was dealing with a tremendous toxic load, which is why

---

18 "How Safe is Splenda? Is Splenda Bad for You?" *MNT*, last updated May 29, 2015, http://www.medicalnewstoday.com/articles/262475.php.

putting me on more medications was never going to solve my health crisis. Resetting my health was the only option that was going to be successful.

Monosodium Glutamate (MSG)

When most people think of MSG, they think of Chinese food. But MSG is hidden in a lot of different foods. Studies have shown that humans are five times more sensitive to this neurotoxin than a rat is. We have glutamate receptors on every major organ, hardwired into our brains, and even on the tip of our tongue. Our bodies are incredibly sensitive to these neurotoxins.

Glutamate is one of the main neurotransmitters for the hypothalamus. As you will learn in Chapter 5 the hypothalamus controls most of our hormones, eating, behavior, temperature control, pain regulation, and sleep habits, as well as the autonomic control of our heart, GI tract, lungs, and bladder. When animals are fed MSG early in life, they develop severe abnormalities—including short stature, small endocrine organs (pituitary, adrenal glands, thyroid, ovaries, testes, and pancreas), and a higher risk of seizures and impaired learning.

Other names for MSG include the following:

- Anything "hydrolyzed," such as hydrolyzed vegetable protein
- Textured vegetable protein
- Yeast extract and yeast food
- Glutamate
- Glutamic acid
- Monopotassium glutamate
- Calcium caseinate
- Sodium caseinate
- Gelatin
- Soy protein, soy protein isolate, and soy protein concentrate
- Whey protein, whey protein concentrate, and whey protein isolate (except approved whey proteins listed at Resetfactor.com)
- Carrageenan
- Bouillon
- Natural flavors or flavoring

- Maltodextrin
- Citric acid
- Anything "ultrapasteurized"
- Barley malt

- Pectin
- Malt extract
- Soy sauce

ACETOMINOPHEN

While many drugs—both over-the-counter and prescription—are toxic to the liver, excessive acetaminophen ingestion is a leading cause of liver failure. Brands like Tylenol, Anacin-3, Arthritis Pain Formula Aspirin-Free, Datril Liquiprin Children's Elixir, and St. Joseph Aspirin-Free Fever Reducer for Children are often used to ease a headache or reduce a fever. However, more than 15 grams of acetaminophen can lead to irreversible liver disease in adults.

The toxic effects of acetaminophen are accelerated by alcohol use. Chronic acetaminophen use and chronic alcohol abuse have been separately linked to kidney and liver disease, according to Dr. Martin Zand, medical director of the kidney and pancreas transplant programs at the University of Rochester Medical Center in New York. If you want to give your liver a break, avoid acetaminophen. If you don't want to destroy your liver cells, never mix acetaminophen with alcohol.

NUTRIENT STORAGE

The last thing to know about this amazing organ called the liver is that it is a huge storage place for many nutrients. The liver can store large amounts of glucose, vitamins, essential nutrients, and minerals. Copper, iron, fat-soluble vitamins (vitamins A, K, E, and D), and vitamin B12 are stored in the liver to ensure that there is always a ready supply in times of need. Fatty acids are also stored in liver tissues.

If you continually damage this organ, you'll deplete the nutrients in it. This will accelerate aging and disease, and it will rapidly break down your body. If you feel as if you're aging fast and not as healthy as you were a few years ago, it may be time for a detox.

This is why the 45-Day Reset starts you with the 15-Day GI and Liver Detox. I can teach you how to eat better and how to stop engaging in harmful food habits that destroy your body, but you have to take the proper steps to repair the damage that is already done. I have found that if you start with a detox and then move into the 30-Day Habit Reset, you'll have results that will last a lifetime.

FRANK AND MARIANA'S STORY

Frank and Mariana both came to me in declining health. They had been living the typical American lifestyle: eating a poor diet, taking multiple medications, and experiencing numerous aches and pains that were only getting worse. Being in their late sixties and early seventies, they assumed that all of this was just the way their health was supposed to be as they got older.

Then their daughter-in-law was diagnosed with stage 4 lung cancer. Looking for lifestyle solutions to her weakened immune system, she applied the principles that we teach in my office. As her health started to improve, it inspired Frank and Marian to see how they could improve their own health.

When I ran an Organic Acids Test on them, I found multiple vitamin deficiencies, depleted glutathione levels, and a growing number of bad bacteria in their guts. I immediately put them on the 15-Day Detox. Within days, weight started falling off them. In 15 days, Frank lost close to 30 pounds, and the aches in his knees and ankles that had been there for years completely went away. Mariana, who had made diet changes prior to her 15-Day

---

Detox, lost 10 pounds, and her energy went through the roof. As I'm writing this, they are 20 days into their 45-Day Reset. Both of them feel and look younger than they have in years. Mariana has lost 29 pounds, while Frank has lost 39 pounds—all in 20 days!

What was the key to their success? What I love about these two is that they were willing to try anything to improve their health. They took my recommendations and followed them exactly. Making food changes, taking supplements to support their liver and gut, and working out for the first time in years was not easy—but the rewards were great.

The other key to their success was that they did it together. I strongly feel that the key to resetting your health is support from the people around you. Frank and Mariana are committed. First, they're committed to themselves. The greatest gift you can give yourself is the gift of health. Second, they're committed to each other. Your health affects the people you love the most. When you're in pain, feeling bad about yourself, or tired all the time, who do you take it out on? Unfortunately, the ones you love the most. When you turn your health around, all your relationships improve. The greatest gift you can give your loved ones is the healthiest you possible.

That's exactly the gift Frank and Mariana gave each other.

CHAPTER 5

Calories Don't Count—Hormones Do

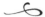

*The doctor of the future will give no medication but will
interest his patients in the care of the human frame,
diet, and in the cause and prevention of disease.*

—Thomas A. Edison

I HAVE GREAT NEWS FOR you! Weight loss is not an issue of eating too much food. It's a hormonal issue.

The only problem is that the hormonal system is complicated. It's like a symphony with lots of pieces that need to be balanced in order for things to work right. There are also lots of toxic influences that break down our hormones. Yet once you understand how all the pieces work together and how you can control these hormones, your body will release weight naturally.

Sound too good to be true? I promise you it's not. In this chapter, I'm going to walk you through understanding hormones. We'll break down the two systems that control hormones (brain and gut) so you can start to understand the underlying cause of your hormonal issues.

Let's begin.

THE BRAIN AND NERVOUS SYSTEM

Hormone production is initiated in an area of the brain called your *hypothalamus*. Chemicals from the hypothalamus get sent to the pituitary, which coordinates all your endocrine glands. The endocrine glands then release the proper hormones needed to do their predesigned jobs in the body.

But what happens if one of your endocrine glands is weakened? Let's use your adrenal glands as an example. When your brain perceives a stressful situation, the hypothalamus initiates the release of a chemical that contacts the pituitary, which in turn releases a chemical to the adrenals telling the adrenals to release the hormone cortisol. Cortisol then moves through your bloodstream, setting off a series of reactions telling the body to get prepared because a stressful event is happening. This is called a fight-or-flight response.

If the adrenals are weakened, the cascade of messages will still get initiated by the brain but the organ receiving the information will be ill equipped to respond. This is what happens with people who are adrenal fatigued. Once a person's adrenals begin to weaken, stressful situations still happen but the adrenals don't produce enough chemicals to give that person the energy needed to handle the stress. The brain still perceives stress and tries to send messages to the adrenals, but the adrenals are too exhausted and don't have the ability to react. Once the adrenals are exhausted, there's not a drug or supplement that will magically turn them back on. The system has to be reset.

One of my patients, Roseen, came to me in a severe state of chronic fatigue. She had tried everything. A mother of two teen boys with a very active lifestyle, she was desperate for a solution. Instead of treating her chronic fatigue, I went searching for the breakdowns. I immediately thought of her adrenal glands.

Before I made any changes to her diet, we worked to strengthen the communication from her brain to her adrenals. It turned out that she had severe damage to her spine. Her spinal curves had all straightened out, and this was causing her nervous system to weaken. Improper communication from her brain, mixed with years of stress, had made her adrenals ill equipped to produce the hormones necessary to give her energy.

We worked on strengthening her nervous system by getting her spinal curves back. Within weeks of corrective chiropractic care, her energy started to come back. Then we added in diet changes, repaired her gut, and pulled toxins out of her body. It took a lot of work and effort on her part, but within months she had dropped over 30 pounds and was beginning to feel like her old self again.

When resetting your health, there's no magic bullet. This is why taking a pill will fail every time. You may resolve an issue temporarily, but if you don't search for how the body got out of balance in the first place, you'll find other systems beginning to break.

I have found that keeping the communication from your brain to your endocrine glands working at 100 percent efficiency is one of the key steps in keeping your hormones balanced. In an earlier chapter, I talked about how the brainstem and spinal cord have a protective mechanism built in to make sure that communication to the organs is happening properly. That protective mechanism is called your spine. Think of the spine as bony armor that helps prevent damage to this important system. The spine was designed to have curves. As a result of the way we use modern day technology—sitting long hours at computers, for example— we're losing these curves. When you lose the curves in your spine, you damage your spinal cord. When you damage the spinal cord, you reduce the amount of information all the organs can receive from the brain.

The thyroid is an endocrine gland that is especially sensitive to changes in the spinal curves because it's located at the base of your neck. The mechanics of a straight cervical spine put a tremendous amount of pressure on the nerves that exit at the base of the neck (at the C5/C6 level). These happen to be the nerves that supply your thyroid.

Among the many studies demonstrating the link between the thyroid and the spine is one in the *Journal of the American Osteopathic Association* that reported a correlation between cervical spine problems and thyroid abnormalities.[19] If you want to balance your hormones permanently, you need to consider your spinal curves. I'll give you more solutions to this

---

19   Murray R. Berkowitz, "Resolution of Hypothyroidism After Correction of Somatovisceral Reflex Dysfunction by Refusion of the Cervical Spine," *The Journal of the American Osteopathic Association* 115 (January 2015): 46–49. doi:10.7556/jaoa.2015.007

in Chapter 7: "Why Your Spine and Nervous System Are Your Fast Pass to Health."

The Gastrointestinal System

Hormones are also made in the gut and liver. A good example of a hormone that is dramatically influenced by the health of the gut is *serotonin*. Simply put, serotonin is a hormone that, when it goes to the brain, makes you happy. Like I mentioned in Chapter 2: "Your Gut Instincts Are Right," over 80 percent of serotonin is manufactured in the gut.[20] When your gut is out of balance, you stop producing the correct amount of serotonin, and that can make you feel depressed.

Research is beginning to show us that there is a connection between serotonin levels and the *type* of good bacteria you have in your gut. An article in Scientific American noted that if certain good bacteria were not present in the gut, your body would not produce the proper amount of serotonin.[21]

As you can see, keeping your microbiome well balanced is also key to keeping your body producing the proper hormonal balance. Once your gut's bacterial balance goes off, your body stops producing the proper hormones to keep you both physically and mentally healthy.

Important Hormones

Although every hormone is important, I want to highlight a few key players: cortisol, estrogen, growth hormone, insulin, leptin, and thyroid. These are the hormones that, if they go out of balance, have the greatest impact on your health.

---

20 "Serotonin," *Wikipedia*, last modified October 30, 2015, https://en.wikipedia.org/wiki/Serotonin/

21 Adam Hadhazy, "Think Twice: How the Gut's 'Second Brain' Influences Mood and Well-Being," *Scientific American*, February 12, 2010, http://www.scientificamerican.com/article/gut-second-brain/

CORTISOL

When they think of cortisol, many people immediately think of the infomercial that advertises the supplement that helps get rid of belly fat that builds due to an increase of stress. And yes, this is exactly what happens when you have too much cortisol surging through your bloodstream. Cortisol levels are directly proportional to stress levels. If you're one of those people who have trouble losing weight, especially around the belly, there's a great chance that your cortisol levels are too high.

Cortisol is secreted by the adrenals. When you perceive something as stressful, the brain immediately sends a signal to the adrenals and tells it to secrete cortisol. The more stress you are under, the higher your cortisol levels. Scientists have known for years that elevated cortisol levels interfere with learning and memory; lower immune function and bone density; and increased weight gain, blood pressure, cholesterol, and heart disease. Chronic stress and elevated cortisol levels also increase risk for depression, mental illness, and lower life expectancy. At least two separate studies have been published implicating elevated cortisol levels as a potential trigger for mental illness and decreased resilience—especially in adolescence.[22]

This is a hormone that you do not want a lot of. There are ways you can naturally lower your cortisol levels. Exercise is one of those ways. This is why in your 45-Day Reset I have you doing Surge Training, which will help your body use cortisol better. A meditation practice will also give you the tools to slow your thoughts down, allowing you to be less reactive to stress and thus further minimizing your cortisol levels. And remind yourself that all stress is self-inflicted and that you can control your reaction to any stressful situation.

---

22 A. Herane Vives et al., "The Relationship Between Cortisol, Stress and Psychiatric Illness: New Insights Using Hair Analysis," *Journal of Psychiatric Research* 70, November (2007): 38–49; S. M. Staufenbiel et al., "Hair Cortisol, Stress Exposure, and Mental Health in Humans: A Systematic Review," *Psychoneuroendocriology* 38, no. 8 (2013): 1220-235.

ESTROGEN

Estrogen is a powerful hormone in both men and women. Estrogen balance is essential for achieving and maintaining fat loss and for preventing diseases like breast cancer. When you have too much estrogen in your body, a condition called *estrogen dominance* can wreak havoc on you both mentally and physically. It can cause you to gain weight for no particular reason, retain water, and feel bloated. It can make you irritable, cause you to feel anxious, give you acne and skin rashes, and create a host of other health and wellness issues. In women, with stress and age, there is a natural decline in testosterone and progesterone levels, leaving a relative excess of estrogen. Fixing estrogen dominance is crucial to balancing all your other hormones.

What causes estrogen dominance? There are only two ways to accumulate excess estrogen in the body: we either produce too much of it on our own or we acquire it from our environment or diet. Unfortunately, accumulating estrogen is not hard. We are constantly exposed to estrogen-like compounds. The most common ways to get estrogen mimickers in your body is through food, beauty products, and plastics. We call these externally sourced estrogens *xenoestrogens.*

When these xenoestrogens enter your blood stream, they attach to estrogen receptor sites, where they block the action of natural estrogen. These estrogen mimickers are one of the major causes of hormonal imbalances in both men and women today. Some conditions currently being linked to an increase in xenoestrogens are infertility, low sperm count, breast cancer, obesity, polycystic ovary symptom (PCOS), and severe perimenopause and menopausal symptoms.

How do you know where you're getting these xenoestrogens from? The Environmental Working Group (EWG), an organization working hard to bring this information to the public, has a list of the most harmful *endocrine disruptors* (another name for mimickers or xenoestrogens). You can find that list at http://www.ewg.org/research/dirty-dozen-list-endocrine-disruptors.

Your best defense against xenoestrogens is knowledge. Start looking for areas that you may be getting these harmful chemicals from. Your beauty products are a great place to start. The EWG also has an app, called Skin Deep, that you can download to help you understand which of your beauty products will disrupt your health the most.

Growth Hormone

If I told you there was a pill that would slow down aging, give you more energy, and turn you into a fat-burning machine, would you take it? Well, there is such a chemical. It's called *growth hormone*. Consider it your fountain-of-youth hormone. The only challenge is that your body stops secreting it in large amounts after the age of 30. That means you have to coax your body into making more growth hormone.

There are two ways to do that.

1. Build more muscle

Many people are focused on staying thin by going straight to a cardio workout at the gym. But I have news for you. If you want to raise your metabolism and improve secretion of growth hormone, you need to build more muscle. Running for an hour on the treadmill will not accomplish that.

One of my favorite ways to improve muscle strength is through resistance training, where you use your body weight *as* weight (as opposed to something external, like dumbbells). Yoga is a good example of this. Many of the poses in yoga strengthen you as you move through your practice. Another great way I like to do resistance training is using an innovative product called a TRX; simple yellow straps that hang from overhead and allow you to do a variety of exercises. You can find these in many gyms and online.

2. Surge Training

If you want the best-bang-for-your-buck workout, Surge Training (otherwise known has high-intensity interval training) is the most helpful workout for weight loss and promotion of health. When you put your body through a series of exercises that cause your heart rate to go up and down, you force your body to secrete growth hormone. I go over how to do a Surge workout in Chapter 11, "The 30-Day Habit Reset."

INSULIN

Want the secret to losing weight? It's regulating this hormone. The best way to regulate this hormone is by decreasing your sugar intake. It's that simple. The challenge you will find is that sugar is everywhere. It's also incredibly addictive. So you need a strategy to get off it. That is one reason why I start your 45-Day Reset with a 15-Day Detox—designed to help you beat this sugar addiction fast.

When we went fat-free as a country years ago, the food industry started increasing the amount of sugar in our foods. Unfortunately, this changed our taste buds and caused most Americans to become addicted to sugar without even realizing it. Every time you eat a food that's high in sugar, your body has to secrete insulin. When secreted by the pancreas, insulin will attach itself to the sugar molecules in your bloodstream and make them usable for energy. When you ingest large amounts of sugar day after day, your body stops reading insulin effectively and you become insulin resistant. This is leading to the growing number of cases of obesity and diabetes in our country.

The CDC estimates that one-third of adults in the United States are now obese, and according to the World Health Organization, almost 40 percent of all adults over 18 worldwide are overweight.[23] Obesity has been linked to many chronic diseases. In fact, according to the National Cancer Institute, obesity is associated with increased risks of several different types of cancer, including colon, breast and thyroid.[24] The estimated number of cases of cancer attributed to obesity is thought to be at least 20 percent. The great news is the same analysis shows that certain

---

23 World Health Organization, "Obesity and Overweight," Fact Sheet no. 311, updated January 2015, http://www.who.int/mediacentre/factsheets/fs311/en/
24 National Cancer Institute, "Obesity and Cancer Risk," http://www.cancer.gov/about-cancer/causes-prevention/risk/obesity/obesity-fact-sheet/

cancers, like breast cancer, can be reduced by as much as 50 percent with a loss of weight of 10kg or more.[25]

A projection of the future health and economic burden of obesity in 2030 estimated that continuation of existing trends in obesity will lead to about 500,000 additional cases of cancer in the United States by 2030.[26] This analysis also found that if every adult reduced their Body Mass Index (BMI) by 1 percent, which would be equivalent to a weight loss of roughly 2.2 pounds for an adult of average weight, it would actually result in the avoidance of about one hundred thousand new cases of cancer.

Have I got your attention? Getting your body out of insulin resistance can save your life. One of the reasons I came up with a 15-Day Detox plan was that I needed to give patients a tool that would kick them out of insulin resistance quickly. During this detox, you will pull all sugar out of your diet and teach your body how to read insulin again.

LEPTIN

In the 1990s, researchers discovered an amazing hormone called leptin. Leptin gets released from fat cells and tells the brain to burn energy from fat. When this was first discovered, researchers thought they had found the cure for obesity and decided to manufacture a pill that simulated leptin. What they found was just like what happens with insulin: people who were holding on to too much weight were leptin resistant. Their brains were unable to read the leptin due to the leptin receptors being blocked.

What blocks leptin receptors? Scientists have discovered that several things block these receptors, but the main foods that block leptin are

---

25 Giovanni De Pergola and Franco Silvestris, "Obesity as a Major Risk Factor for Cancer," *Journal of Obesity* 291546 (2013).

26 California Assembly Committee on Health, "Subject: Women's Health," http://www.leginfo.ca.gov/pub/15-16/bill/asm/ab_0951-1000/ab_990_cfa_20150425_125528_asm_comm.html.

toxic processed foods. Anything with partially hydrogenated oils in it will clog these receptors and make your body hold on to fat no matter what you do. I've found that when people are trying to lose weight and can't seem to drop a pound no matter what they try, they are leptin- and insulin- resistant. You have to address those issues first if you want to lose weight. Depriving yourself of calories or hopping on a treadmill for hours won't do it. The 45-Day Reset is designed to reset both these hormones.

THYROID HORMONES

From this point forward, whenever you think of your thyroid, I want you to think of your gut and the spinal curves in your neck. Just like the studies done on neck curves and the function of your thyroid, there is a strong correlation between our thyroid function and the health of our gut. Your thyroid might be able to secrete enough T3, T4, and TSH, but it needs healthy bacteria in the gut to be readily available so that those hormones can be absorbed. Eating probiotic-rich foods or taking a high-quality probiotic will help your body be better equipped to absorb these key thyroid hormones.

If you have signs of thyroid problems—such as unexplained weight gain, cold hands and feet, depression, or hair loss—yet your blood tests are all showing normal thyroid hormone levels, look at the microbiome of your gut. If the microbiome is off, your body may not be absorbing thyroid hormones properly.

Your thyroid is also highly susceptible to toxins. If you have read this far in the book, you know we live in an extremely toxic world. One way to protect against the toxins that destroy the thyroid is to take an iodine supplement. Many experts feel that the toxins in our environment have depleted our natural iodine stores. The thyroid needs iodine to function normally. Since many people are walking around with a deficiency in this key mineral, taking an iodine supplement will help build the thyroid strong and help protect it from all the toxic exposure.

FIONA'S STORY

Fiona has been a patient of mine for years. She always has an upbeat spirit and a can-do attitude that serves her well in life. Despite this great attitude, her health was not thriving, and it was starting to affect her life in many ways. I helped her to reset her metabolism by balancing her hormones through diet changes, repairing her gut, and strengthening her nervous system. The results were not only profound, they have been lasting. Her story is best told in her own words:

Despite living what I thought was a fairly healthy lifestyle, my health was not getting better. In fact, it was getting worse. My digestion was not great. I was getting to the point where I had gas daily. I was also having headaches a couple of times a week. I'm an athlete, and it seemed the more I practiced, the more weight I gained (and it wasn't all muscle). And I always seemed to be tired. I was also beginning to develop seasonal allergies. Finally, I had acne, no matter what I tried, and I've always had a reddish color to my face.

My poor health was affecting my performance as an athlete. I had very little energy and endurance. My allergies were starting to affect my job as a counselor. I was having trouble talking without coughing. For my allergies, I tried a variety of over-the-counter medicines and relied on cough drops a lot; they worked with varying effectiveness, but nothing worked really well. For my acne, I tried all sorts of products over the years, but none of them seemed to make much of a difference.

The hardest part about the diet changes Dr. Mindy recommended was the sugar withdrawal. I craved things that I don't even usually eat! However, I found that being able to eat good fats helped. Eating good fats satisfied my sugar cravings in a way that was actually more satisfying than if I'd had the sugars. It was also difficult cutting most carbs and grains from my diet, but when compensated for with the good fats and other great recipes Dr. Mindy provided me, I found that I was more satisfied. As a lazy cook, I also found myself cooking more. I was enjoying cooking more because I knew that what I was making was going to taste great.

The results came slower for me because it probably took me about a month to get the hang of the diet. But almost right away, my digestion improved and the amount of gas I had decreased significantly. I also noticed that my skin started to clear up, including the redness that I never even thought was abnormal. I started losing weight as well.

The results I got with the 45-Day Reset Program have been mind-blowing for me. I have lost around 25 pounds. People I didn't even know commented on how much weight I had lost. Some people even told me to stop or that they hadn't thought I had that much to lose in the first place. More importantly, I have gained health that I never even knew was nutrition related.

I now have clear skin and great digestion with no gas. I no longer have headaches. My seasonal allergies are gone. I am no longer tired all the time, and I no longer get tired after eating and/or in the late afternoon. However, my absolute favorite result is that with no sugar in my body, I have no muscle burn when training in my sport! This alone has caused my endurance to skyrocket and has improved the quality of my performance overall. I have won the National Championships since changing my nutrition, and I give credit for that to the 45-Day Reset Program.

Furthermore, now when I eat things not on the nutrition plan, very few of them are as satisfying (either in taste or in physical satisfaction) as I remember them being. I also typically feel bad after eating something off the plan. I have a lack of energy and returned symptoms (especially poor digestion and acne), and I even get emotional and sometimes depressed. Now I am much more selective when I eat things that are off the Reset Factor nutrition plans.

My advice to people wanting to reset their health is to stick with it and not give up or beat themselves up when their discipline fails! It's OK to not be perfectly strict all the time! It's going to happen—just move on when it does.

Doing the 45-Day Reset, even if you're not perfect, will make a huge difference in your health! Also, when you're struggling to make a healthy decision versus an unhealthy decision, take your focus off the negative (such as all the things you're not getting) and instead keep it on how great you're going to feel when you're healthier and how satisfying and tasty the things you can eat are.

CHAPTER 6

Reclaim Your Birthright—Power Up Your Own Natural Immunity

Natural forces within us are the true healers of disease.

—Hippocrates

MOST PEOPLE HAVE NEVER BEEN taught how miraculous their own immune system can be. You were built with an internal medicine cabinet inside you, capable of fighting foreign invaders such as bacteria, viruses, and fungus. Your immune system is also designed to recognize cancer cells and destroy them. It's an incredible aspect of your body, and if you keep it strong, it can protect you from even the strongest of infections.

Learning how to maximize this system is key to staying healthy all year round. In this chapter, we'll look at some of the amazing things that your immune system does for you. We'll also look at why the immune system breaks down and what you can do to strengthen rather than weaken your wonderful immune system.

WHAT'S A FEVER?

Stop and think for a minute why your body would raise its temperature. It must be trying to burn something out, like an infection. A fever is a beautiful gift—a natural way to destroy bacteria and viruses. Yet what do most people do when they first feel their temperature rise? They take a pill to lower it. This can damage your body's natural healing mechanism and leave your body wide open for the infection to keep growing. This is why, while you will often feel better when you take a Tylenol or Excedrin to lower the fever, once the drug is out of your system, your body will want to raise its temperature again—because it still has an infection to kill.

You'll notice throughout this book that I'm trying to give you the tools to read your body. These tools will help you reset your body back to its original design. The more toxins you put into your body, the less it will function the way you want it to. Taking medications for every uncomfortable feeling we have in our body does not strengthen it. In fact, it weakens it.

So what can you do when you have a fever—other than taking medication? My advice is to think about how you can assist your body. It has decided to raise its temperature to burn an infection, so what can you do to help it burn that infection? Put an extra layer of clothes on. Lie on the couch and rest. Drink lots of fluids. Take a probiotic to increase the good bacteria going into your gut.

But be sure to monitor your fever. Keep it under 105 and everything should be fine. One of the most frequent and unnecessary visits to the emergency room is for fevers that are not at a dangerous temperature.

What About Mucus or a Cough?

Mucus is something everyone has—and some people wish they had a lot less of the stringy, gooey stuff. Sure, it can be gross to blow globs of snot into tissue after tissue when you have a cold or sinus infection, but mucus actually serves a very important purpose.

"Mucus is incredibly important for our bodies," explains Michael M. Johns, III, MD, director of the Emory Voice Center and assistant professor of otolaryngology (head and neck surgery) at Emory University. "It is the oil in the engine. Without mucus, the engine seizes."

How much mucus is normal, and how much is too much? What does its color tell you about your health? Can you just get rid of it or at least cut down on it—and how should you do that? These are all great questions. In order to answer them, it's important to first understand what mucus is doing for you.

What is the mission of mucus? Mucus-producing tissue lines the mouth, nose, sinuses, throat, lungs, and gastrointestinal tract. Mucus acts as a protective blanket over these surfaces, preventing the tissue underneath from drying out. "You have to keep them moist, otherwise they'll get dry and crack, and you'll have a chink in the armor," says Neil L. Kao, MD, associate professor of medicine at the University of South Carolina School of Medicine.

Mucus also acts as a sort of flypaper, trapping unwanted substances like bacteria and dust before they can get into the body—particularly the sensitive airways. "You want to keep that environment, which is a sterile environment, free of gook," says Dr. Johns. "Mucus is kind of sticky and thick. It's got viscosity to it that will trap things."

But mucus is more than just sticky goo. It also contains antibodies that help the body recognize invaders like bacteria and viruses, enzymes that kill the invaders the mucus traps, and proteins to make the mucus gooey, stringy—and very inhospitable.

Sounds like a pretty helpful mechanism, right? Well, then, why would you want to kill this mechanism by taking an antihistamine? No, it's not fun to have sinus pain. But if you could remind yourself that it's serving a key purpose, then you might be able to hang in there a bit longer with your nose running.

If you're one of those people who constantly have sinus problems, the key is to get to the root of *why* your body is producing so much mucus. A good reset to your body, especially your gut, will often address the breakdowns that are causing your body to produce mucus in the first place.

WHAT ELSE DOES MY IMMUNE SYSTEM DO?

When it comes to your immune system, most people think its main purpose is to fight infections. But with the growing number of toxins in our environment, the larger concern for the immune system these days is fighting cancer cells. Most people don't want to think about this, but the reality is that you have thousands of cancer cells inside you right now. In fact, as you're reading this, your brain is identifying where these cells are and how to get rid of them. Hopefully, you have a high-functioning immune system that is identifying and killing those cells.

According to Dr. William Li, MD, cancer researcher, president, and medical director of the Agiogenesis Foundation, all it takes is for one of the trillions of cells inside you to mutate for a cancer cell to be born. Dr. Li says that you don't get cancer like you catch a cold. You provoke a healthy cell, and it mutates into a cancer cell.

What would provoke a healthy cell to mutate? There are a variety of reasons, but a diet packed with sugar and chemicals would be a good prime suspect. Once a cell mutates into a cancer cell, it's your immune system's job to identify the foreign cell and kill it. With most people eating the standard American diet—packed with inflammatory, acidic foods—many people are living in a body that is too acidic. Your immune system is weakened by an acidic environment. A weak immune system will not fight cancer well. A key part of building a strong immune system is getting your body back to the alkaline side, as it was designed to be.

WHAT IS ALKALINITY?

A big part of resetting your health is rebuilding your body at the cellular level. As I mentioned before, our body has seventy-two trillion cells, all of which have to be coordinated correctly to make sure our bodies function properly. The cells have a *pH level* inside them. In 1931, Dr. Otto Warburg, won the Nobel Peace Prize for his discovery that every person who had cancer had an acidic cellular pH. He went on to say that cancer cannot thrive in an alkaline, high-oxygen environment.

What are the mechanisms behind the cell's pH level? Inside every cell is a *mitochondrion*. One of the key processes that mitochondria are responsible for is the production of ATP—the molecules that give you energy. The more ATP you have surging through your body, the better every system will work—including your immune system—and the more energy you'll have.

In order for a mitochondrion to produce energy, it needs the inside of the cell to be alkaline. If the internal environment is not alkaline, then instead of producing ATP, a mitochondrion produces lactic acid. Cancer thrives in a lactic acid environment. One of the reasons cancer patients are so low in energy is that their cells are producing lactic acid instead of ATP.

How Do You Keep Your Body on the Alkaline Side?

The first step to being alkaline is understanding what your cells' pH level is right now. You can easily find pH strips online or at your local health food store or pool supply store. Follow the instructions and monitor your pH. The healthiest pH to be at is 7.4. If you really want to be as accurate as possible, get the pH strips that test your urine. Be sure to test first morning urine, as that will give you the best reading.

Once you have identified what your pH level is, the fastest path to improving your pH is by adding greens into your diet. I make it a personal pledge to have greens with every meal. Parsley, all lettuces, cucumber, and avocados are great quick-and-easy ways to slip some greens into your meals without having to make a whole salad.

The other fast way to alkalize your body is by juicing, especially with green juice. With a high-quality masticating juicer, you can drink your greens and alkalinize your system quickly. When you remove the fiber of the green vegetable and concentrate the nutrients in a juice form, it makes it extremely accessible to your cells.

Many people look at their medicine cabinet as the place they store key items that keep them healthy. I actually don't believe that health lives there. Medications like Tylenol, Excedrin, Claritin, and Nyquil might be in your cabinet to give you symptom relief when you're sick, but they do not promote health. In fact, they often destroy your health. I believe that the best medicine cabinet consists of the tools in your kitchen. The two tools I believe every house should have are a blender and a juicer.

Blenders are fantastic for making smoothies, which you will see in your 45-Day Reset. What I love about smoothies is that if you combine the proper ingredients, you can literally get all the nutrients you need to be healthy for a day. I put as many of my supplements, veggies, and healthy foods in my smoothie as possible. This way I know I'm set for the day. You'll find some of my favorite smoothie recipes at the back of this book.

Drinking smoothies is also a phenomenal way to get high-quality nutrition into your kids. Both my kids are very active. Often, I'll see them in the morning and not again until night. They both get a smoothie for breakfast because I want to make sure they get all the nutrients they need for the day.

Juices made with a high-quality juicer are exceptional at quickly moving your body into an alkaline state. The best juicer is a masticating one. It's a bit more expensive, but it's worth the money. Masticating juicers extract the nutrients from foods in a way that allows the cells of your body to use those nutrients more effectively.

The other word for *masticating* is *cold-pressed*. You can find cold-pressed juices at most grocery stores. If you're buying juice at a grocery store, be sure it is cold-pressed because juices that aren't give you no nutritional benefit.

How Do I Tell Which Juice Is Best?

As I mentioned above, cold-pressed juice is what you want. It will cost you more money, but in my opinion, it's the only kind to buy for your health. Other juices may taste great but add no benefit to your pH. Many people are buying juice at the store thinking that it will make them healthier, when in reality, it's doing the opposite.

Sugar content is another thing to be aware of when you're buying juice. Many people like the taste of higher-sugared fruits like mangoes, bananas, and pineapples. When you go to buy a juice at the store, your taste buds will want those. But if you want to change your pH, you need a low-sugar, high-green juice. Always look at the sugar amount on the nutritional label and stick to the lower-sugar juices.

When you're sick, you may reach for the orange juice, hoping it will build your immunity. Although vitamin C is fantastic for your immunity, buying orange juice is not the answer. First, orange juice is extremely high in sugar. Too much sugar in your body suppresses your immune system. Orange juice is also acidic and will create an acidic environment inside your cells. You're better off buying a low-sugar green juice to alkalinize your body and taking a vitamin C supplement.

WHAT BREAKS DOWN YOUR IMMUNE SYSTEM?
You may be surprised how easy it is make certain lifestyle choices that will begin to break down your immunity. These choices impact the health of your gastrointestinal system, your nervous system, and the other systems of your body. The following are the main insults to your immune system:

YOUR STRESS
Everyone knows that stress is harmful to the body. Unfortunately, the system that stress often hurts the most is the immune system. How does this happen?

When you're chronically stressed, your body secretes more cortisol. *Cortisol,* which we talked about in an earlier chapter, is a chemical that suppresses inflammation during a response to stress. If it's present in the blood for long periods, the body develops a resistance to cortisol and does not respond to it properly. Instead, the body ramps up production of substances that actually promote inflammation, leading to a state of chronic inflammation.

These pro-inflammatory substances, called *cytokines*, are associated with a host of chronic inflammatory and autoimmune conditions. Autoimmune conditions occur when the body basically mistakes itself as a threat and attacks itself. Examples are fibromyalgia, rheumatoid arthritis, and lupus. Other chronic conditions affected by this chronic stress reaction include diabetes, heart disease, and cancer.

Chronic stress suppresses critical pieces of our immune system. This makes the body susceptible to acute illnesses and prolonged healing times. *Lymphocytes* are an example of one of the immune cells that are lowered during times of stress. Lymphocytes are a major component of the immune system. They kill invading organisms that would cause disease and they recognize harmful substances and help defend against them. Cortisol and corticosteroids suppress lymphocytes. With a lowered number of lymphocytes, the body is at increased risk of infection and disease.

YOUR NUTRITION

Nutrition involves more than just choosing what tastes good. You truly are what you eat. A diet high in toxins, inflammatory foods, sugar, and processed foods will not only promote inflammation but will also make you acidic. The standard American diet is packed with these foods, and that is one of the many things that has led to increased cancer rates in our country. The other damaging effect of these foods is that they kill the good bacteria in your gut. You need good bacteria to kill infections that enter the digestive system.

As I mentioned in Chapter 2, your gut is key to producing many essential vitamins. If you're deficient in those vitamins because your gut is damaged, your immune system will not work properly. Think of vitamins like the fuel in your car. If you don't have the right fuel or enough fuel, your car will not function properly. The challenge with a poor diet is not only that it damages healthy bacteria but that as that damage persists, it also makes you deficient in key vitamins.

This is why resetting your immune system has to include resetting your gut.

A study at Harvard Medical School found a relationship between good bacteria and the immune system.[27] It's now known that certain bacteria in the gut influence the development of aspects of the immune system, such as its ability to correct deficiencies and increase the numbers of certain T-cells. T-cells are crucial for identifying and destroying viruses, bacteria, and fungi. Avoiding highly processed foods and adding in a high-quality probiotic are good habits to implement to strengthen your immunity.

One of the greatest ways you can suppress your immune system is by eating sugar. Linus Pauling, who helped discover the amazing benefits of vitamin C for the immune system, felt that reducing sugar should be part of your immune protocol. Consuming sugar and refined carbohydrates effectively crowds out vitamin C and prevents it from entering the cells.

Researchers at Huntsman Cancer Institute in Utah also discovered that sugar feeds tumors. According to the Institute, "It's been known since 1923 that tumor cells use a lot more glucose than normal cells." In fact, it's been found that there are six times as many insulin receptors in specimens of breast cancers than are found in healthy breasts.[28] This is why when your doctor wants to see if you have cancer, he or she will order a PET scan. PET scans involve giving the patient a glucose mixture intravenously or via a drink or injection. Cancer cells absorb glucose more quickly than do other cells, so giving the patient a glucose mixture makes cancer cells easier to identify on the scan. Why would all those cancer cells come out? Because they love sugar. The more sugar you eat, the happier your cancer cells become.

---

27 Hachung Chung et al., "Gut Immune Maturation Depends on Colonization with a Host-Specific Microbiota," *Cell* 149, no. 7 (2012): 1578–93, http://www.sciencedirect.com/science/article/pii/S0092867412006290/

28 V. Papa et al., "Elevated Insulin Receptor Content in Human Breast Cancer," *Journal of Clinical Investigation* 86, no. 5 (1990): 1503–10, http://www.ncbi.nlm.nih.gov/pmc/articles/PMC296896/

YOUR TOXIC LOAD

The number of toxins you are exposed to every day also has a large impact on your immunity. The toxins in your food leave your small intestine and go directly to your liver, which plays a major part in your immune system as the body's main organ of detoxification. Your body is designed to detoxify itself. However, when external sources of toxicity are added to the mix, normal detoxification processes become overwhelmed.

A fully functional liver supports immune system function. If your liver is preoccupied with the demands of detoxing, it will not give your immune system the support it needs. This will leave you wide open to infections.

Toxins are also now considered a major contributor to many cancers. As we discussed in Chapter 4, the liver is one of the most important organs in the body. An increase in toxins will put a strain on it and ultimately leave it depleted, overworked, and unable to keep up with the demands that have been placed on it.

On average, we Americans consume fourteen pounds each year of food additives—including colorings, preservatives, flavorings, emulsifiers, humectants, and antimicrobials. We also consume on average one pound of pesticides and herbicides each year, according to the book *Digestive Wellness* by Elizabeth Lipski, MS, CNN. In 1990, the EPA estimated that seventy thousand chemicals are commonly used in pesticides, foods, and prescription drugs. The use of pesticides and herbicides to limit crop loss has skyrocketed over the past thirty years, and our toxic load is higher than at any other time in history.

We've talked a great deal about the effects of toxins as related to other organs and systems. The other damaging effect of toxins is that they create *free radicals*. Free radicals damage normal healthy cells and bind to immune cells, damaging immune pathways. Because of their damaging effects to the immune system, free radicals have long been associated with the ability of cancer cells to multiply in the body. A diet high in processed foods and low in fruits and vegetables will increase the amount of free radical damage in your body.

Toxins are not only prevalent in your food—you'll also find them in your beauty products and household products. The increase in the number of medications prescribed has also increased the toxic load of many Americans. And your skin is the largest organ of your body. Whatever you put on it will be directly absorbed into your bloodstream and will go directly to your liver.

The path to health has to be easy and time efficient or else you won't follow it, and trying to identify which products are highly toxic to your body can be a daunting task. But with their Skin Deep app (http://www. ewg.org/skindeep/), the Environmental Working Group has made it easier to identify which beauty products are highly toxic and which are OK. Download it onto your phone and be sure to check all your lotions, shampoos, gels, makeup, and anything else that goes onto your skin or hair. You want those products to score a 3 or below on the Skin Deep app.

YOUR SPINE AND DAMAGE TO YOUR NERVOUS SYSTEM

Many of you may be surprised to find your spine listed in this chapter on the immune system. The spine protects the most important organ in the human body—your nervous system. Anything that damages your spine will damage your nervous system.

When your nervous system gets damaged, the communication from the brain to your body will be altered. Your spine was designed to be in a very specific place. When the vertebra in the spine shift out of this place due to physical, emotional, and chemical stress, a variety of health problems can occur. Numerous studies have demonstrated how restoring proper alignment of the spine can improve your immune function. I will go through those studies in detail in Chapter 7, "Why Your Spine and Nervous System Are Your Fast Pass to Health."

YOUR SLEEP LEVELS

As I mentioned in Chapter 3, sleep is how your body repairs itself. You need a good night's sleep to keep your immune system functioning at its best. According to Diwakar Balachandran, MD, director of the Sleep Center at the University of Texas M.D. Anderson Cancer Center in Houston, several studies show our T-cells go down if we're sleep deprived. He also states that inflammatory cytokines go up from a lack of sleep, leaving us at greater risk for colds and flus. In simple terms, sleep deprivation suppresses the immune system. The more all-nighters you pull, the more likely you are to decrease your body's ability to respond to colds or bacterial infections.

My general recommendations when you feel a cold coming on are to cut out the sugar, increase the raw greens, take probiotics and vitamin C, get your spine adjusted, remove all toxic food from your diet, and sleep. Your body will heal. It was designed to fight infections.

NADIA'S STORY

A few years ago, a patient came to me having been diagnosed with breast cancer. She was only 30 years old and the mother of two young children. For three years she had been on intense chemotherapy. But despite all medical attempts, the cancer was growing. She was given months to live. Scared and feeling hopeless, she came to my office as a last resort to see what she could do to strengthen her immune system naturally.

I immediately changed her diet, taught her how to identify known carcinogens in her home and beauty products, and gave her strategies to strengthen her immune system through supplements, chiropractic care, and stress management. Our goal was not to treat the cancer but to create an environment inside her that was unfavorable to cancer growth.

Much like what the doctors did for me when I had chronic fatigue, we created a multipronged approach to building health from the inside out. Within four months, she had dropped 30 pounds. Her energy and spirits were up. She was feeling better than she had in years.

When she went for her first PET scan since changing her lifestyle, they found that for the first time since she had been diagnosed, the cancer wasn't getting worse and in some areas the cancer cells were shrinking. Something had stopped it from growing. We were encouraged. She continued on her new healthy path and within a year, the tumors began to shrink. At the time of writing this book, there is only one area in her body where cancer still exists. Her body's immune system has kicked into high gear and has slowed down the cancer's ability to multiply.

To me, the surprising part of Nadia's story is how little information she was given on what she could do on her own to help strengthen her immune system. She desperately needed a reset—but she was given only medication. Once we identified where her immune system was broken and repaired those breaks, her immune system started finding cancer cells and killing them.

PATTY'S STORY

When Patty was diagnosed with breast cancer, she sought traditional medical treatment. And it worked. Relieved that she was able to overcome this scary disease, Patty went back to living life as she had before cancer.

A relative of hers recommended she read a book called *Cancer Killers,* by Dr. Charles Majors. It's the story of how one man reversed several brain tumors by identifying what caused his cancer cells. At the time, Patty was feeling secure and happy that she had beaten cancer; she had no expectations of the cancer coming back.

But it did. Several years later, her cancer returned. This time it was in her lungs. Doctors told her it was stage 4 and gave her months to live. In a panic, Patty dusted off her *Cancer Killer* book and started voraciously reading about how her body had built cancer.

I met Patty soon after that. We immediately changed her diet, started corrective chiropractic care, and worked on repairing her gut and strengthening her immune system with supplements. Like Nadia, she chose to do both conventional and natural health care treatments. Patty was incredibly strict with the foods she ate, making sure that she didn't eat anything that would feed the cancer. Within months, the cancer began to disappear. Her doctors were shocked. Within less than a year, the tumors had completely disappeared.

Nadia and Patty are amazing examples of how powerful the immune system can be. The health plan they followed in my office was not geared toward treating cancer. It was aimed at strengthening their bodies so cancer could no longer exist within them. Like Dr. Li mentioned above, cancer cells are mutations of normal healthy cells. When you stop creating an environment that causes the cells to mutate, cancer will stop growing.

In the third section of this book, I will go deeply into the mindset of health. When Nadia and Patty made the decision to reset their health, they had to change their mindset from "a pill is going to cure me" to "I have the power to beat this." The same goes for you. Many of you reading this book may be in a really tough state of health. Some of the ideas in this book may be overwhelming, radical, and against what society has taught you about health. Be open. The minute you change your mind from being a victim of your condition to being the victor over your circumstances, you will begin to heal.

That's what both Nadia and Patty did. Instead of hoping the miracle cure would show up, they put themselves into action—and not just a little action. They changed everything about their lifestyles. They looked at any behavior they had that might have provoked a normal cell to mutate into a cancer cell. They reset their health.

I love the term *reset* because that is what so many people need. With so many toxins in our lives, it's easy to get off course. But you have the power to change that. You have the power to reset your health whenever you choose. You get to be the boss of your health. You just need to be willing to let go of old beliefs and health habits that may not be serving you anymore. Once you do, there is a whole new healthy world waiting for you.

CHAPTER 7

Why Your Spine and Nervous System Are Your Fast Pass to Health

Look well to the spine for the cause of disease.

—Hippocrates

HAVE YOU EVER BEEN TO Disneyland? If you have, you know that the key to speeding up the wait in line is a Fast Pass. Well, your body has a fast pass to healing: it's called your spine and nervous system. Taking great care of your spine speeds up the function of your nervous system. Unfortunately, by now you've probably noticed a common theme in this book: our bodies have been destroyed by the modern conveniences of the world we live in today. Nowhere is this more apparent than with our spine and posture.

The ironic thing is the fact that in many cases, toxins were originally developed to make our life easier. I'm sure that the first time a toxin like partially hydrogenated oil was put into a food product, consumers were excited that it extended the shelf life of that food. That made the food more convenient and minimized how often people needed to go to the store—a quick, satisfying solution to the problem of not having enough time. But over time, we've come to realize that processed foods such as partially hydrogenated oils may be more convenient but are also destroying our health.

The same thing is now happening with technology and our posture. Using smartphones, laptops, and tablets has made life much easier for us—but unfortunately, it's also destroying our posture. It would be one thing if our posture were just an issue of looking good, but there is growing evidence that poor posture equals poor health. Not only are foods and toxins destroying our guts, leading to imbalances in our brains, but posture can dramatically affect how well our brain and nervous system function.

So what can you do about it? We'll discuss this problem and some solutions in this chapter. First, we'll look at how your brain communicates with your body and how the way you use modern technology is changing the curves in your spine. Next, we'll talk about how you can identify whether your spine has problems. Finally, we'll talk about the potential of corrective chiropractic for realigning your spinal curves and removing the cause of many imbalances in your body.

The good news is that if you're aware of a problem with your posture, you can change it. Remember, our body always wants to go back to its original design. It just needs a strategy to do so.

How Your Brain Communicates with Your Body

How many of you have ever thought about your spinal cord? Probably not many. But your spinal cord is one of the most important parts of your body. It has one job: to let information flow in and out of your brain.

When you look at how the spine was designed, looking at it from the side, it was meant to have curves. Those curves are there to protect the spinal cord. The spinal cord is the only path by which the brain can send information to the other parts of the body. In men, the spinal cord is usually 18 inches long, and in women, it's 17 inches long. And it needs to be relaxed in order for the messages from the brain to be sent clearly.

So what happens if you sit at a computer all day? You take out these curves and put them in a completely reversed position, stretching the spine to new and unfamiliar lengths. And what if you do that day in and day out for decades? Do you think it's possible to do that and keep your normal curves over time? The answer is no. We are seeing more and more evidence of people losing the natural, normal curves in their spine—and the damage is becoming irreversible.

Orthopedic surgeons have now come up with terms they call *text neck* and *forward head posture* (FHP) to identify these spinal changes. The number of cases of adolescents and young adults needing disc surgery in the lower cervical spine is growing due to the increase in habitual forward head position.

But that is only a small part of the damaged being done by the stretching of the spinal cord. Researchers are also noticing that because of the importance of the upper cervical spine to the brain's communication with the respiratory and digestive systems, people who have FHP also have slower digestive tracts and are getting less oxygen in and out of their lungs. Changes in your posture are no joke!

Here's how your brain communicates. At the top of the spinal cord sits your brainstem. When your brain sends a signal to the cells of the body, the information flows in and out of the brainstem. The brainstem acts as a connection from your brain to your spinal cord. It carries life-sustaining information, serving as the center of control over vasomotor, respiratory, and cardiac functioning. It also plays a part in digestion. It is such an important part of our brain that we have very special vertebrae designed to protect it: the *atlas* and *axis.*

Christopher Reeve learned the importance of this neural area when he was in a horse accident that fractured both his atlas and axis. When his upper cervical vertebra broke, it jammed right into his spinal cord. Because this area carries information that controls digestion and respiration, his digestion and lungs immediately stopped functioning. The pressure from those bones on the brainstem was so traumatic, the brain couldn't get the information to those organs to make sure they were functioning properly.

One growing concern is that we too are damaging these two bones that protect our brainstem. With our constant use of cell phones, tablets, and laptops, we spend hours every day with our heads flexed forward. This is causing an unusual amount of pressure on our brainstem and spinal cord and is impairing the flow of information that coordinates digestion, respiration, and the production of hormones like serotonin. Although this damage is not as initially traumatic as the damage that Christopher Reeve endured, the long-term effects are very similar to the symptoms he had.

What are the harmful effects of FHP? More and more doctors are addressing these damages to the spine. Rene Cailliet, MD, director of the Department of Physical Medicine and Rehabilitation at the University of Southern California, wrote about its effects in his book *The Rejuvenation Strategy*:

Incorrect head positioning leads to improper spinal function. The head in forward posture can add up to thirty pounds of abnormal leverage on the cervical spine. Forward head posture results in loss of vital lung capacity. In fact, lung capacity is depleted by as much as 30 percent. Loss of lung capacity leads to heart and blood vascular problems. The entire gastrointestinal system is affected, particularly the large intestine. Loss of good bowel peristaltic function and evacuation is a common condition that comes with forward head posture and loss of spinal lordotic curves.

Forward head posture causes an increase in discomfort and pain. Freedom of motion in the first four cervical vertebrae is a major source of stimuli that causes production of endorphins, like serotonin. Forward head posture causes loss of healthy spine-body motion. The entire body becomes rigid as the range of motion lessens. Soon, one becomes hunched.

WHAT YOU CAN DO?

So what can you do to avoid the debilitating effects of FHP? The first thing is to know what your spinal curves look like. Unfortunately, you can't tell what your spinal curves really look like—whether they're normal or how much damage your spine has—without an X-ray. So if you're not already seeing a chiropractor who specializes in spinal correction, now would be a great time to have your spine looked at.

There are also a couple of tests you can do yourself. Next time you look in the mirror, look at your shoulders and notice whether they're even. Does your head tilt to one side or the other? Look at yourself from the side (using a mirror). Do your ears come forward in front of your shoulders? They should be directly over your shoulders. These are both great examples of the body adapting to the changes in these curves.

Other ways to know if your spinal curves have changed include reading your symptoms. Remember that symptoms are like dashboard lights on your car. When they come on, they're telling you that something is wrong inside your body. Some symptoms of FHP and spinal cord changes include the following:

> Headaches
> Low-back pain
> Neck pain
> Allergies
> Digestive issues
> Immune system challenges

> Fatigue
> Sinus problems
> Ear infections
> Lack of focus
> Hyperactivity, especially in children

Once you have identified that there are imbalances in your curves, a chiropractor can make specific adjustments and give you specialized homecare and rehabilitation exercises that will bring your correct curves back.

Because our children are growing up on technology, I recommend you also do these observation exercises with your children. In my own practice, I'm starting to see these spinal changes at younger and younger ages. A scientific principle known as Wolff's Law states that once your spine has changed from its original design, gravity is so forceful that over time it will start to decay your bones. Very much like a cavity that will rot a tooth, changes in your spine will progress quickly. But just as you can catch a cavity before it rots a tooth by having regular dental checkups, finding changes in spinal curves before the spine decay or scoliosis sets in is always a smart idea.

Remember that the whole goal of the 45-Day Reset is to bring your body back to its original design, turning on your healing capabilities on the inside. If there is damage to your spinal cord and spinal nerves because of changes in your spinal curves, you can feed your body all the great nutrition you want but you still won't be able to repair it completely.

OTHER CAUSES OF IMPROPER SPINAL CURVES

A common question I'm asked is "What causes these curves to change, besides technology?" My answer is to ask more questions: "How do you sit? Do you slouch in your chair? Are you slumped over your computer?" Look at your posture and how you sit the majority of the day and you can start to answer these questions yourself.

Sports injuries also change spinal curves, especially in children. Contact sports—such as football, rugby, basketball, and soccer—all have a propensity to damage the spine in a permanent way. I cannot emphasize enough the benefit of having a good corrective chiropractor on your team to coach you through the daily stresses that destroy the spine and give you a protocol to repair them. Car accidents also create significant damage to your spine. One serious whiplash injury can straighten your cervical curve.

There are a few steps you can do at home to help your spinal curves out. One of my favorite at-home exercises is to take a towel, roll it up, and slip it under your neck and lower back. If you do this at night, before you go to bed, it helps to reset your spine and posture, lengthen the ligaments and muscles, and give your spinal curves a break from the damaging stress of the.

CORRECTING THE SPINE TO STOP DISEASE

Because the nervous system delivers information from the brain to the body and tells injured cells to heal, anything that improves this communication will speed up healing. One reason chiropractic is such a popular form of health care is that when you take pressure off your spinal cord and nerves, your body heals at a significantly faster rate. This is why over 30 million people see a chiropractor every year.

Still, although chiropractors are the most commonly visited doctors other than medical doctors, every once in a while I get someone who says, "I don't believe in chiropractic. Show me the science." Well, multiple studies have been done on the efficacy of chiropractic. Here are some of my favorite ones.

CHIROPRACTIC AND BLOOD PRESSURE

This study watched 25 patients with early-stage high blood pressure over an eight-week period. Their cervical spine was X-rayed, and measurements were taken of the atlas vertebra—the doughnut-like bone at the very top of the spine. Half the group was given a specific chiropractic adjustment, the other half a placebo adjustment. Those who got the real procedure saw an average 14 mmHg greater drop in systolic blood pressure (the top number in a blood pressure count) and an average 8 mmHg greater drop in diastolic blood pressure (the bottom blood pressure number) than the group that got the placebo adjustment.[29]

"This procedure has the effect of not one but two blood-pressure medications given in combination," study leader George Bakris, MD and director of the University of Chicago Hypertension Center, told WebMD. "And it seems to be adverse-event free. We saw no side effects and no problems."

In my own clinic, I have seen many cases where a patient's blood pressure drops just from getting his or her atlas realigned. It makes sense that

---

29 "Special Chiropractic Adjustment Lowers Blood Pressure Among Hypertensive Patients with Misaligned C-1 Vertebra," The University of Chicago: Medicine, March 14, 2007, http://www.uchospitals.edu/news/2007/20070314-atlas.html.

if the atlas is misaligned, it can squeeze the brainstem and cause blood pressure to rise. Remember, the brainstem is one of the most vital parts of the central nervous system. The minute you take pressure off the brainstem, your body can reset itself and your blood pressure will be reduced.

SPINAL CARE AND THE IMMUNE RESPONSE

In his book *The Cancer Killers,* Dr. Charles Majors states that researchers have known for a long time that there's a critical link between the central nervous system and the immune system. During the 1918 flu epidemic, in which more people died than in all wars combined up to the time, it was found that the death rate of chiropractic patients was one-fortieth that of non–chiropractic patients. How did this happen? What does a chiropractic adjustment do for your immune system? And can a chiropractic adjustment have an effect on your cancer- and infection-fighting system?

A 2010 study published in *Chiropractic & Osteopathy* showed that the immune cells that fight cancer respond directly to chiropractic adjustment. One of these immune cells is called interleukin-2. When released into your body, interleukin-2 creates a cascade of events that help your body attack cancer cells and other infections. This study looked at 74 people and monitored their immune response after a thoracic adjustment. What they found was that "chiropractic adjustments temporarily influence interleukin 2-regulated biological response following a single adjustment."[30]

Another study, done by Patricia Brennan, PhD, showed that after receiving an adjustment to the middle back, patients had an increase in their white blood cell count. White blood cells are a critical component of the immune system that fights bacteria, viruses, and fungi. If you don't have enough white blood cells, infection can take over your body. This is one of the challenges cancer patients face: low white blood cell counts.

---

30 Julita A. Teodorczyk-Injeyan, Marion McGregor, Richard Ruegg, and H. Stephen Injeyan, "Interleukin 2-regulated *in vitro* antibody production following a single spinal manipulative treatment in normal subjects," *Chiropractic & Osteopathy* 18, no. 26 (2010): published online, doi:10.1186/1746-1340-18-26

Patients evaluated in this study had their white blood cell count measured pre- and post-adjustment. What Dr. Brennan found was that fifteen minutes after the adjustment, patients had a surge of white blood cells. She concluded that there was an "enhanced respiratory burst" following a chiropractic adjustment.[31] This burst is necessary for our immune cells to destroy unwanted foreign chemicals, invading viruses, and bad bacteria.

Researchers have also looked at the power of chiropractic for AIDS patients. In a person with AIDS, the immune system is losing the battle against a deadly virus. A group of HIV-positive patients were given chiropractic adjustments over a six-month period. The researchers found that the patients who were adjusted had a 48 percent increase in the number of CD4 cells, a powerful immune cell that kills viruses, while those that didn't receive the adjustments experienced a 7.96 percent decline in the number of CD4 cells over the same period.[32]

Finally, a study done by the *Journal of Orthopedic Surgery* researched the possible connection between chronic nerve compression and vertebral deformity in the thoracic region and chronic allergy and asthma problems. It was determined that the adrenal cortex functions of these patients were compromised due to the ongoing nerve compression. When this group was given a chiropractic adjustment to release the nerve pressure, they had a 70 to 80 percent improvement in their condition.[33]

---

31 P. C. Brennan et al, "Enhanced Neutrophil Respiratory Burst as a Biological Marker for Manipulation Forces: Duration of the Effect and Association with Substance P and Tumour Necrosis Factor," *Journal of Manipulative and Physiological Therapeutics* 15, no 2 (1992): 83–89; P. C. Brennan et al., "Enhanced Phagocytic Cell Respiratory Burst Induced by Spinal Manipulation: Potential Role of Substance P," *Journal of Manipulative and Physiological Therapeutics* 14, no. 7 (1991): 399-408.

32 Jeffrey L. Selano, et al: "The Effects of Specific Upper Cervical Adjustments on the CD4 Counts of HIV Positive Patients," *Chiropractic Research Journal* 3, no. 1 (1994).

33 Y. Takeda & S. Arai, "Relationship Between Vertebral Deformities and Allergic Diseases," *The Internet Journal of Orthopedic Surgery* 2, no. 1 (2003).

A Chiropractor on Your Team

Can you see why 30 million people go to a chiropractor every year? Getting pressure off your nervous system is one of the most helpful gifts you can give your body. Pinched nerves are not just an issue of pain. As noted above, you can pinch a nerve and it can slow down your immune response, increase your blood pressure, and eventually cause you pain.

How can you find a great chiropractor? Unfortunately, not all chiropractors are the same. In fact, it is very confusing for the general public to understand the differences between chiropractors. Here are some of the criteria for finding a great chiropractor that I tell friends and family about if they live in other towns:

- A thorough diagnostic evaluation is needed. Look for someone who is thorough with you on your initial visit. In my book, X-rays are key to identifying the changes in your spine.
- Spinal correction is a must. You want someone who will correct your spine. We call this corrective chiropractic. Although powerful, one adjustment can have only a temporary effect. You need a chiropractor with a game plan—someone who will measure your spinal misalignments and create a plan for correcting them.
- You and your chiropractor should be a team. Home exercises, nutritional advice, and strategies for keeping your spine healthy for life should all be a part of your care.

Hopefully, you now have a great understanding of how your body works and where it is breaking down. If you get in the middle of your 45-Day Reset and begin to lose momentum or enthusiasm, pick this book up and re-read one of the chapters in the second section.

I remember when I was pregnant with my first child. Everything was new and unfamiliar. There were days when I would come home from work feeling horrible. It helped tremendously to read books on what was going on in my body at that point in my pregnancy. When I understood the big picture and why my body was feeling the way it did, it lifted me up and helped me get through those hard days.

This book can do the same for you. Knowledge is power. Keep learning how this miraculous body of yours works. Never give up on having amazing health. With the right attitude, a great plan, and a hopeful heart, anything is possible.

Now, let's reset your health!

Part 3

⮂

The 45-Day Reset

CHAPTER 8

Setting Yourself Up for Success

You can't always get what you want. You get what you're committed to.

—Anonymous

As I mentioned in Chapter 3, your greatest weapon in the fight to heal your body is your brain. Not only does your brain control all 72 trillion cells of your body, but it also helps you stay the course. If you train it well, it will keep you disciplined, focused, and motivated as you embark on your 45-day health journey.

Before I walk you through the specifics of your 45-Day Reset, there are a few key strategies I want you to implement to create a winning mindset and set yourself up for success. I also want you to get clear about why you're doing the 45-Day Reset, find an accountability partner, pick the right 45-day period, and be careful whom you talk to. Most important: believe in yourself!

We'll talk about each of these in this chapter.

YOUR "BIG WHY"

I can show you the path to an amazing, healthy life, but I can't motivate you. That's your job. The great news is even if you have failed a thousand times at dieting, you can succeed this time! Here's the trick: you need to be clear from the beginning *why* you're doing it.

Start by thinking about what life would be like if you didn't have extra weight, pain, or disease holding you back. Living in a body that doesn't feel the way you want it to is a major block to living an amazing life. So just think for a moment: what would your life be like if you didn't have your health problems to deal with? Would you be a better parent? Would you be happier in your marriage? Would you be more productive at work? My guess is that the answer to all these questions is probably yes.

I know this because for several years, I lived in a body that felt terrible. I know what it's like not to have enough energy and to feel bad about your weight. It affects *everything* you do. I want you to begin to dream again. I want you to *believe* in yourself again. Just for the next few minutes, think about how awesome life would be without the limitations of your body holding you back. This can be hard at first, because if your body has been broken for a while, you might not even remember what a great-feeling body feels like. But keep dreaming.

Most people aren't aware of the fact that every night when they go to bed, their body is repairing itself. In a seven-year period, you will have a whole new body on a cellular level. This is great news for you! It means you can rebuild your body. I promise you it won't take seven years. If you follow the 45-Day Reset exactly as I lay it out for you, you will be living in a different body in 45 days.

The key to having a successful journey is to want the result you're about to get—badly! You have to want it more than you fear and dislike the obstacles that may present themselves during your 45-Day Reset. The more mentally hungry you are for a change in your health, the more successful you will be at this program.

ACTION STEP #1: WRITE DOWN YOUR "BIG WHY"
Why do you want your health to change? Write down your Big Why on a piece of paper or sticky note. Put this somewhere you can see it on a daily basis: in a journal, in your car, or where you brush your teeth—a place where it will constantly remind you of your dream. Pictures, quotes, and

motivating words to yourself are all great! The key is that they have to stir something emotional inside of you. Your Big Why should fire you up when you think about it.

CHOOSING AN ACCOUNTABILITY PARTNER

Having an accountability partner has been one of the keys to my success with health. One of my best friends is a phenomenal accountability partner. Whenever I start a new workout program or health change, I usually commit to that change for 30 to 45 days. I do that because I know that's how I make a lasting change. I always ask her to be my accountability partner because she makes me believe in myself.

Recently we did a 30-day exercise program together. It was 30 days of exercise for 30 minutes a day. Several days a week, I work 12 to14-hour days. Those are the days I normally don't work out, and I was a little resistant to working out on those days until she reminded me it was just 30 minutes and that I probably spend that much time on social media on those days. She was right. So I committed to myself and to her.

On the second day of the program, I had worked a twelve-hour day; I was exhausted and I did *not* want to exercise. But I had made a commitment to her. I didn't want to let her down—she believed in me, and I didn't want to destroy that belief. I ended up working out and feeling fantastic, and I was so grateful that she was my accountability partner.

You need at least one person to be your accountability partner—someone who knows how badly you want to change. This person needs to have your back and want you to be as healthy as you do. You need to not want to let this person down.

Choose your accountability partner wisely. This person needs to lift you up when you don't want to do the program anymore. He needs to be someone strong enough not to let you off the hook and caring enough that he wants to see you succeed even if his own health is not in a great place. Ideally, as you make changes and people see your results, you should inspire them to want to be better and change themselves. I've seen this happen often: when a patient loses weight, the next thing you know, all the patient's family and friends are on the 45-Day Reset—they want to experience the same results the patient is getting.

Unfortunately, the opposite is also true. Years ago I had a patient who was significantly overweight. Her mother had died of cancer, and she made the decision that she didn't want to follow the same path. She decided to lose weight.

She had a group of friends, also significantly overweight, who were supportive of her and cheered her on. Within months, she lost 40 pounds and was looking and feeling great. But as she dropped her weight, her friends changed from great cheerleaders to unsupportive critics. As she left her work every night to go to the gym, they started making comments like "You're more concerned about losing weight than being home for your children after work." Then, when she stopped going out to restaurants that had the foods she was avoiding, they would remark on how she never hung out with them anymore.

As ugly as it is, sometimes the people closest to you will feel threatened by your success. That is what happened with this woman. Ultimately, her friends brought her self-esteem down, and within a year's time, she had gained all the weight back.

Action Step #2: Pick an Accountability Partner

Tell your accountability partner what you're doing and why. Tell her that you need her love and support, especially on the days you want to go back to your bad habits. Let her know what your goals are for the 45 days you will be following the 45-Day Reset.

Planning for Success

The last thing I want to mention is this: look at what will be going on in your life in the next 45 days. Remember how I mentioned you need to prepare for obstacles. If you think ahead and prepare for these obstacles, they won't take you off course. With this in mind, there are several action steps you can take to set yourself up for success with this program:

1. Pick 45 days that you can commit to. You get what you're committed to, so pick a 45-day period in which you're going to make your health a priority over everything else. I promise you that the way I'm going to teach you to eat is something you can easily follow for life. But when you first make changes, it can seem frustrating. So don't try this on vacation or during an extremely stressful time.

2. Look at your calendar. Do you see any parties, BBQs, or holidays coming up? A one-time event doesn't need to block you from starting the program, but I want you to prepare for it. The first 15 days you're on this program, you will be detoxing. You won't be drinking alcohol or eating sugar, so if there's a party coming up and you know it will be difficult to resist the temptation to consume those things, wait till that event is over to start the program.

Occasionally, a patient tells me there is no 45-day period without a social event. If that is you, don't wait. You may be one of those people for whom the time will never be perfect. The trick is to know when the events are coming up and how to prepare for them. If you're going to your best friend's house for a BBQ, where you know she'll make your favorite meal—which is not on the reset plan—there are a few things you can do.

First, don't go hungry. Eat before you go. We make horrible food choices when we're hungry. Second, bring your own Reset Factor–approved meal. Some people tell me they don't like to stand out and make a fuss. Let me tell you, more people will be interested in and inspired by why you are committing to your health than will criticize you. Third, remember your Big Why. Don't let others steal your dream of being healthy. Yes, certain foods taste amazing. You know what's even more amazing? Living in a body you love!

3. Plan ahead. Before I leave the house every day, I think through what my meals will be and make sure I'll have access to healthy foods. If I know that getting to the right food will be difficult that day, I bring healthy food with me. I often leave the house with a large bag of cut veggies, quinoa salad, and avocado. You will never find me far from a bag of raw almonds, because if my blood sugar starts dropping, I want to have something healthy quickly available so that I can bring it back up. Make sure you have the right foods on hand before you start the program!

BE CAREFUL WHOM YOU TELL

I know this sounds crazy, but as I mentioned before, not everyone wants to see you succeed. And for some reason, when it comes to health, people have strong opinions. Not all these opinions are accurate. I've seen patients who were super gung ho about a 45-Day Reset get shot down in the first week when their spouse told them that all the fuss about sugar is unscientific. Remember, your best weapon for better health is your brain. Not only does it heal you, but it can keep you motivated throughout the 45 days of the Reset. So be careful whose words you let into your brain.

For the next 45 days, you're only going to tell the people in your life whom you feel have your back and want you to succeed. This might require that you hibernate a bit. That's OK. I have done cleanses during which I just had to check out of my social group for a few days until I started feeling strong with my cleanse and my body began craving health more than anything. When your body craves health, it can override your brain. Once you're feeling great and your sugar cravings are gone, a chocolate cake can be placed in front of you and all you will think about is how awesome you feel and how horrible you will feel if you eat that cake.

THE 30-SECOND RULE

This brings me to my last point. I was a huge bread and sweets person for years. When I made the decision to lose weight and put my health first, I had to come up with some tricks to help my brain get past the desire for sweets. So I came up with something I call the 30-second rule.

When something gets placed in front of me that I want to eat but I know won't benefit my health, I first think about how I will feel an hour after I eat that food. Most of us enjoy the immediate gratification of food and don't think ahead about how we'll feel afterward. For some, you will feel physically bad. But for many of you, it may not be a physical pain but a mental one. You will feel bad about yourself, frustrated that you are failing at another diet, and discouraged with yourself.

I then remind myself that when I taste that food, it will taste amazing for about thirty seconds. In my opinion, that is a very short time of gratification in exchange for hours of feeling bad. It's not a worthy exchange, if you ask me. So next time you feel like eating something off your 45-day plan, ask yourself if it's worth it.

BELIEVE IN YOURSELF

I believe in you. I know what the human body is capable of. I have watched thousands of people bring their health back following the path you are about to start. Each one of those people had a unique set of challenges and hurdles to get over. Each one wanted health badly and was willing to achieve the goal at all costs. You are no different. You can achieve the same results! You just have to believe in yourself, stay committed to yourself and the program, and follow the path outlined for you. If you do, you will succeed!

CHAPTER 9

The Reset Truths of Health

Nothing tastes as good as healthy feels.

—Anthony Robbins

THERE ARE EIGHT KEYS TO health that have the power to dramatically influence the way you feel and function in life. I call these *reset truths* because they are absolutes when it comes to changing your health habits. If you pay attention to these principles, you will be successful. I recommend you continue to observe these truths even after you finish the 45-Day Reset, as they're simply good health principles to follow.

The body needs three things to heal: time, repetition, and energy. The reason I have you do this program for 45 days is that you need enough *time* to give your body a chance to get rid of injured cells and make healthy new ones. *Repetition* is key because every day that you follow your new health habits, you build momentum. The more you stick to the program, the easier it gets. And the more *energy* you put into this program, the more you will get out of it. Try new recipes in the back of the book. Go explore a farmers' market in your area. Make it fun. At the end of the 45-Day Reset, you will feel like a new person.

Let's look now at the eight reset truths of health. Applying these truths to your life will put you on the road to health even before you start your reset!

1. Labels Tell a Story

For the next 45 days, I want you to read every label you come in contact with. If you're going to eat it, I want you to know what's in it. The golden rule for label reading is that if you can't pronounce a word in the list of ingredients, it's probably a chemical. The following are a few of the key ingredients you want to stay away from:

Butylated Hydroxyanisole (BHA)

BHA is a synthetic antioxidant used to inhibit oxidation of fats and oils in food, thereby preventing rancidity. But by keeping your food from going bad, BHA may in turn be putting your body at risk. Some studies have shown that BHA causes cancer in animals, and it's anticipated that it may be a human carcinogen. Try to avoid BHA and look for foods that use vitamin E as an antioxidant instead.

Butylated Hydroxytoluene (BHT)

Like BHA, BHT is used to prevent oils in food from going bad. It's commonly found in many cereals to preserve freshness. BHT has been found to increase hyperactivity in children, and laboratory results have found that it increased the risk of cancer in animals as well. Like BHA, BHT should be avoided whenever possible.

Sodium Nitrite and Sodium Nitrate

Nitrites and nitrates are commonly found in foods such as hot dogs, lunch meats, and bacon because they help the meat retain its color and prevent bacteria formation. They can lead to the formation of cancer-causing chemicals, so it's best to avoid any packaged foods that contain these preservatives. Several studies have linked increased sodium nitrite intake from hot dog consumption to childhood leukemia. You want to avoid these preservatives at all costs.

POTASSIUM BROMATE

Commonly found in bread and baked goods, potassium bromate is used to strengthen dough and lower baking time, but it has been found to cause kidney and nervous system disorders, cancer, and gastrointestinal issues.

HYDROGENATED OILS

Hydrogenated fat, also known as trans fat, is created by converting liquid vegetable oils into solid fat through a hydrogenation process. These oils raise your bad cholesterol, lower your good cholesterol, interfere with your body's ability to fight cancer, and increase your risk of heart disease. These synthetic fats are found in many snack foods and desserts.

Recently, the FDA issued a declaration of intent to ban hydrogenated and partially hydrogenated oils from all foods. According to the statement, these fats are "unfit for human consumption." They stated that by 2018, these harmful fats must be completely removed from all food products.[34]

TERT-BUTYLHYDROQUINONE (TBHQ)

TBHQ is added to foods (especially animal fats) to help extend their storage life. Also used in other products such as cosmetics, TBHQ can cause nausea and possibly increase your risk of cancer. Although it may be tolerable in low doses, try not to eat too many foods that contain this ingredient to prevent possible side effects.

2. EATING FRESH FOOD IS BEST

Fresh food is anything that has a short shelf life. When you walk into a grocery store, the fresh food is around the perimeter of the store. Vegetables, fruits, and meats are great examples of fresh food, and every meal you eat

---

34   U.S. Food and Drug Administration, "FDA News Release: The FDA Takes Step to Remove Artificial Trans Fats in Processed Foods," last updated June 16, 2015, http://www.fda.gov/NewsEvents/Newsroom/PressAnnouncements/ucm451237.htm.

needs to have plenty of fresh items. This does mean going to the store more often, but I promise you it's worth it. Fresh live foods like vegetables build health. They have enzymes in them that are crucial to your digestion.

You need to be eating one pound (approximately two cups) of fresh vegetables a day. Not only is this a great way to get more vitamins and minerals into your body but the fiber will help pull toxins from your body.

3. EATING FAKE FOOD WILL MAKE YOU SICK

Once you develop the habit of reading labels, stop eating fake food. *Fake food* is anything that is laden with chemicals and that has been altered from the original food itself. Potato chips are a good example of this. A potato is healthy. A potato chip has chemicals in it and is fake. Fresh cheese with no added ingredients is real food; Velveeta cheese has been altered with chemicals to make it taste different and last longer. Butter is a real food; margarine is a fake one. Another term for fake foods is *processed foods*. Anything that has been altered from its original natural state potentially has harmful chemicals in it.

If you have trouble deciding whether a food is fake or not, ask yourself whether nature made this food or whether it was made by humans? Because processed foods have become so prevalent in recent years, you can also ask yourself if the food you are about to eat was available when your grandmother was a child. The presence of chemicals in our food is a recent phenomenon. Our grandparents were not exposed to the toxic foods we're now exposed to. Fresh apple pie is definitely something Grandma would have made. A prepackaged Hostess apple tart? Probably not in Grandma's diet.

4. YOUR BODY NEEDS WATER

Seventy percent of our body is made up of water. This makes water the most important nutrient you need. Yet most people don't drink enough. A well-hydrated body is crucial to optimal health. Dehydration can lead to fatigue, headaches, wrinkles, suppression of the immune system, and low back pain. Most people don't realize that often when you're hungry, it's actually your body being thirsty.

The best way to add more water into your body is to start your day off with a glass of water. What you put in your stomach first thing upon rising is absorbed into your body the quickest. This is why I recommend the detox water during your 15-Day Detox (see Recipes section). Make sure to always have water with you—at your desk, in your car, on the countertop in your kitchen. Six to eight glasses a day is a best practice. Room temperature water is easiest on your digestion. You can add fresh organic lemon juice for added detoxifying benefits.

5. Sugar Stops Your Body from Burning Fat

The fastest way to destroy your metabolism is to eat a diet high in sugar. It has been well documented that cancer cells have a higher number of receptor sites for sugar, which enables them to easily use glucose as a food source. Sugar has been known to increase inflammation in the body and raise your blood pressure, and it's now considered a major contributor to cardiovascular disease. Plus, a diet high in sugar will cause your body to become insulin resistant and force you to pack on pounds quicker than anything else.

You'll notice as you go into your 15-Day Detox and 30-Day Habit Reset that I have you take sugar out of your diet completely. For many of you, this will be challenging but one of the most rewarding experiences you'll ever have.

Sugar is hidden in almost every food in your grocery store, so make sure to read those labels. Look for anything that ends in *–ose,* as that is most likely sugar.

Here is a list of common words for the sugar in your food that you want to avoid:

- Agave nectar syrup
- Barley malt
- Beet sugar
- Brown-rice syrup

- Brown sugar
- Cane juice (evaporated or not) or cane sugar
- Caramel or caramel coloring
- Corn sweetener
- Corn syrup or corn syrup solids
- Date sugar
- Dehydrated cane juice
- Dextrin
- Dextrose
- Diastatic malt
- Fructose
- Fruit juice
- Fruit juice concentrate
- Galactose
- Glucose
- High-fructose corn syrup
- Honey
- Invert sugar
- Lactose
- Malt syrup
- Maltodextrin
- Maltose
- Mannitol
- Maple syrup
- Molasses
- Palm sugar
- Raw sugar
- Rice bran syrup
- Saccharose
- Sorbitol
- Sorghum or sorghum syrup
- Sucrose
- Syrup
- Treacle
- Turbinado sugar
- Xylose

If you see any of these words on your labels, avoid them.

The other way to know what sugar is in a food source is by reading the nutrition label. Stop going to the calories and go straight to the sugar content. The American Heart Association says that men should have no more than 35g and women no more than 25g of sugar daily, so when you read your label, start by counting the sugar. To give you some examples, a Jamba Juice smoothie has 48g of sugar, a vitamin water has 41g of sugar, and a Coca-Cola has a whopping 91g of sugar.

In the 1970s, our country declared a war on heart disease and the food industry took all fat out of many products we had access to—leaving many foods tasteless. So to improve the taste, the food industry has slowly increased the amounts of sugar in foods. You will find that sugar is in almost everything, so pay close attention.

In a study published in 2007, M. Lenair, F. Serre, L. Cantin, and S.H. Ahmed showed that our brains are actually more addicted to sugar than to chemical stimulants like cocaine.[35] Every time you eat sugar, the chemical dopamine is released into your bloodstream, making you feel euphoric. This is why you keep going back for more. But your pancreas can't keep up with the amount of sugar you're giving it, so it eventually wears out. This increase in sugar consumption is why diabetes is affecting more Americans today than ever before.

The *glycemic index* measures the sugar content of food and how it affects your glucose-insulin levels. The higher the number on the index, the more damaging the sugar. To give you some perspective, refined sugar has a glycemic index of 100. Honey has one of 55, coconut sugar has one of 30, and stevia and xylitol have a glycemic index of 0. This means that when you digest stevia and xylitol, they will not allow your pancreas to secrete insulin or your blood sugar to increase in any way, shape, or form.

You'll notice in the recipe section that many of the recipes call for these lower-indexed sugars. Many people may find the taste of stevia and xylitol artificial even though they are natural substances, so try coconut sugar as it has a lower glycemic index and is often more pleasurable to the taste buds. This is the one sugar that I find my kids will accept, and we no longer have any other types of sugar in the house. The beautiful thing about coconut sugar is that it has a 1–1 ratio with cane sugar, so any recipe that calls for a cup of sugar can be replaced with a cup of coconut sugar. It's that easy!

---

35 Magalie Lenoir, Fuschia Serre, Lauriane Cantin, and Serge H. Ahmed, "Intense Sweetness Surpasses Cocaine Reward," *PLOS ONE* 2, no. 8 (2007): doi:10.1371/journal. pone.0000698

6. You Need Good Oils to Burn Fat

I have shocking news for you! We are one of the most fat-deprived nations. Your body needs fat to perform any crucial function, like making good cholesterol, nourishing the brain, and metabolizing fat. Yes—most people don't realize that *you need fat to burn fat.*

One key step to living a healthier life is understanding that not all fats are created equal. There are good fats and there are bad fats. You absolutely want to pull bad fats out of your diet. In fact, one of the worst fats is partially hydrogenated oil.

The list below contains the bad fats you need to pull out of your diet immediately:

- Hydrogenated and partially hydrogenated oils
- Rancid oils (corn oil, vegetable oil, canola oil, cottonseed oil, soybean oil, safflower oil, and sunflower oil)
- Trans fats (margarine, synthetic butters, and shortening)
- Roasted nuts and seeds
- Roasted nut and seed butters
- Pasteurized and homogenized dairy products

Consumption of bad fats promotes the following diseases:

- Arthritis
- Type 2 diabetes
- Autoimmune diseases
- Neurological diseases
- Alzheimer's disease
- Cancer
- Cardiovascular disease
- Pulmonary disease

Good fats on the other hand, will promote health. Good fats to add into your diet are the following:

- Oils: coconut oil, avocado oil, olive oil (cook on medium heat only), walnut oil, flaxseed oil, hemp seed oil, and grapeseed oil

- Animal proteins: grass-fed meat, wild fish (especially wild salmon), organic cage-free eggs (pasture-raised is best)
- Dairy: Full-fat raw milk (whole or cream), raw cheeses, organic butter, ghee, and kefir (without sugar added)
- Other: olives, avocados, and any coconut products (milk, butter, flakes, flour, flesh, etc.)

Your body thrives on good fat. Your brain needs fat to function properly. Good fat is known to lower your triglycerides, increase your metabolism, and improve your mental health—and it's now strongly being linked to helping your body fight cancer.

A patient of mine was really suffering with her health. She was on several medications and in constant pain, and her doctor was really on her to change her diet to improve her LDL and triglyceride levels. She had been doing low-fat dieting for years, but these numbers were not changing. She had also had no luck at losing weight. Once she did the 45-Day Reset with us, her triglyceride levels lowered and weight starting falling off of her. Her body desperately needed good fat to function properly.

As sugar is taken out of your diet, you might find that your hunger temporarily increases. The key to making sure that this does not happen is to increase these good fats. In fact, right now, many of the healthiest diets, such as the Paleo or ketogenic diet, have people obtaining 40 to 70 percent of their calories from fat. This is why you'll see that in your 15-Day Detox, when we have you drinking smoothies, we have you add in coconut oil. This will help curb your appetite, nourish your brain, and speed up your metabolism.

7. Go Organic

As I explained earlier in this book, most health problems are toxicity issues. One of the most common places to get toxins in your diet is from the chemicals sprayed on fruits and vegetables, as well as the chemicals that are injected into the animals we eat. No one is free from the over-spraying of our food.

It's time for you to start taking those chemicals out of your diet. The first step I recommend is going organic with your meats. It's become common practice to add growth hormone and antibiotics to cows and chickens before they're slaughtered and made available for human consumption. Those chemicals will definitely get into your body and destroy your good gut bacteria.

When you're at the grocery store, look for meats that say "no added hormones or antibiotics" and "organically raised." These chemicals are becoming so well known as destroyers of our health that even companies like Tyson Chicken are starting to pull them from their food products.

The other food you want to minimize because of its toxic load is pork. The pig is the one animal that does not have a sweat gland, and thus it retains all of its toxins inside the fat. When you eat pork, you get a high dose of extremely toxic meat. Even when it's organic, it should be ingested in moderation.

Once you have gone organic with your meats, go organic with your fruits and vegetables. If you're worried about the cost of organic food, here a some things to think about. First, the most expensive way to take care of your health is to ignore these steps and wait for a medical crisis. It is much cheaper to pay for your health now, as opposed to paying for a medical crisis later. Something as simple as switching over to organic fruits and veggies could save you thousands of dollars down the road in medical bills. So change your mind set on how you look at cost savings as it pertains to your health.

A good general rule to follow is this: everything on the EWG's Dirty Dozen list should be bought organic. For things on the Clean Fifteen list, such as avocados (which are ridiculously expensive when bought organic), you can get away with buying nonorganic. You will find that list in the 30-Day Habit Reset chapter. A general guideline for eating organic is meats first; once you have accomplished that, fruits and veggies second.

8. Just Say No to GMO

I have mentioned GMOs in several places in this book. I can't emphasize enough how toxic GMO food is for your health. Avoid it at all costs, as it will destroy your gut. During your 45-Day Reset, you will take all GMO food out of your diet.

How do you know if it's GMO? Unfortunately, America's labeling laws around GMOs are minimal. Some foods are well-labeled and some are not. Since my number-one reset truth is "read labels," you should be able to identify whether a food is organic or not by looking at the label. Anything with a label that says "USDA Organic" on it will be GMO-free. Some products go as far as putting an actual "Non-GMO" label on the package. If you see both of those labels, that's great! If you see none of these labels, you may be eating a food that has been genetically modified.

Here are the most commonly genetically modified crops:

- Corn (field and sweet)
- Soybeans
- Cotton
- Canola (another reason to avoid this harmful fat)
- Alfalfa
- Sugar beets (this means refined sugar as well)
- Hawaiian papaya
- Squash

9. Make Dinner Your Lightest Carbohydrate Meal

For those of you who want to lose weight, the fastest way to pack on the pounds is to eat the majority of your calories after dinner—especially calories that come from carbohydrates. What happens to most people is this: They come home at the end of a day and eat a large carbohydrate-filled meal, complete with alcohol and a dessert. This causes their insulin to spike so high that it doesn't come down before they go to sleep. All that extra insulin while you're sleeping will turn to fat. In fact, sumo wrestlers know this quite well, and because one of the demands of their sport is to add on weight, their training regime includes eating a carbohydrate meal and then taking a nap.

So if you're interested in losing weight, one of my top recommendations is that your largest meals should be breakfast and lunch, and dinner should be your lightest meal with the least amount of carbohydrates. The only exception to this is if you decide to do intermittent fasting (see Chapter 11). You never want to go to sleep with a full stomach of undigested food and high insulin counts in your bloodstream. Because of this, many of my patients who do the 15-Day Detox choose to eat their one meal at lunch, not dinner. This gives their body time to digest the food and use the insulin well before bedtime.

Not eating late poses a problem for a lot of people because, like you, they have conditioned their body to desire something sweet after dinner. The first thing you have to realize is that this is just a habit you've created—it's not that your body actually needs it. My dad is a really good example of that. As a child, he was always given a bowl of ice cream after dinner. Although he ate extremely healthy, 70 years later he still has trouble breaking that habit because it is so ingrained in him. Be sure to look in our recipe section for desserts you can eat that will satisfy your sweet tooth but not spike your insulin levels.

When people come to me and want to lose weight, my first recommendation is this: no fruits, alcohol, breads, or pastas after 3:00 p.m. A dinner high in protein and veggies on a consistent basis will have you losing weight faster than a sugar-free treat laden with chemicals for dessert.

Overwhelmed yet? If you read these rules and wanted to put the book down, hold on! This will be easier than you think. Because the 45-Day Reset is geared to teach your body to crave health more than the treats you've become accustomed to, all you have to do is take the first step. Trust the program. I can't tell you how many of my patients think the 45 days is going to be grueling and take a whole lot of willpower—then come back to me and tell me how easy it has been. The same will be true for you.

Now that you understand these basic truths about health, you're ready to get started. In the next chapter, we'll start the 15-Day GI and Liver Detox program.

CHAPTER 10

The 15-Day GI and Liver Detox

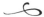

I'VE TRIED EVERY DETOX ON the planet myself. I've starved myself, drunk funky shakes, taken massive amounts of herbs, done colonics, enzyme baths, and wraps. I've eaten only fruits and vegetables for weeks on end. One cleanse consisted of ten days on only lemon, cayenne, and maple syrup. Although many of these approaches made me feel great at the time, the re-entry back to food was difficult, and I found that within a few months, I felt worse than ever before.

But I've finally learned how to detox right, and that's what I'll share with you now. This detox will provide your body with the many benefits of cleansing, support your gut to regrow healthy bacteria, cleanse your liver, and leave you looking and feeling radiant. As you know by now, I call it the 15-Day GI and Liver Detox, or the 15-Day Detox for short.

In this chapter, I'll share all the steps of the 15-Day Detox with you: what you'll need, what the daily program looks like, and what to expect day to day. I'll start with my top tips for a smooth detox and end by answering frequently asked questions.

RESET DETOX TIPS

In order to make sure you get the most out of your detox, here are my top tips

Keep in mind that many popular detox protocols are just a pause button that gives your liver a small break from the toxic load it's under.

You don't do enough to heal the liver and gut. Once the detox is over, you go back to your old habits, you start to gain weight back, and eventually you go right back where you started—feeling horrible. In fact, I've watched many people have a rebound effect after they detox. They're so happy that the detox is over, they eat more of the harmful foods they love and gain *more* weight back.

I don't want that to happen to you. So let's make sure you do this right by carefully reading through the following reset detox tips and the guidelines for the 15-Day Detox.

RESET DETOX TIP #1: KNOW WHY YOU'RE DETOXING

Remember your Big Why? Knowing it for your detox is key to your success over the next 15 days. The first few days of a detox can be tough, so being connected to your Big Why will help. If permanent weight loss is your goal, the 15-Day Detox is a perfect starting point.

Not sure if you need a detox? Here are some of the warning signs your body will give you that it's time to detox:

- ➢ Feeling stressed
- ➢ Mood swings and headache
- ➢ White- or yellow-coated tongue and/or bad breath
- ➢ Fluid retention and/or congested sinuses
- ➢ Increased belly or visceral fat
- ➢ Cravings and/or blood sugar issues
- ➢ Gallbladder issues (or you've had your gallbladder removed)
- ➢ Abdominal bloating
- ➢ Overheating/excess sweating
- ➢ Weight loss resistance
- ➢ Acne, rosacea, itchy skin
- ➢ Fatigue unrelieved by more sleep, especially in the morning
- ➢ Moodiness
- ➢ Autoimmunity
- ➢ Chemical sensitivity (You're a lightweight when you drink alcohol, or smelling fragrances makes you anxious.)

> ➤ Insomnia, especially early morning awakenings such as 1:00 a.m. to 4:00 a.m.

> ➤ Cravings, especially for sugar, alcohol, and refined carbohydrates

If you have four or more of these signs, you may have a congested liver that needs some help.

Reset Detox Tip #2: Don't Starve Yourself

Many people mistakenly believe that in order to provide a proper detox for their bodies, they need to starve themselves. Nothing could be further from the truth. Your body needs nutrients to heal and cleanse itself. Starving yourself for an extended period of time puts undue stress on your liver. This is why you need a thorough detox strategy that gives your body all the nutrients it needs to repair itself.

You'll notice in the 15-Day Detox that you're given the option to eat throughout the day. Just by eating the right things, your body will cleanse and regenerate naturally. I want you to eat enough good food to flood your liver with nutrients while pulling out the toxins. Detoxing done right is the greatest way to rebuild a healthy liver and reset your metabolism for good.

Reset Detox Tip #3: Start by Repairing Your Gut

If there is a breakdown in your gut, such as leaky gut syndrome, you'll overtax your liver with too many toxins. Once the liver gets flooded with toxins, it stops metabolizing fat. Anytime you want to reset your metabolism, you need to repair the gut and get nutrients to the liver to help it break down fat again. This is why during your 15-Day Detox, you'll start by repairing your gut and liver.

I recommend you use a high-quality, high-powered probiotic during your entire 45-Day Reset. Most people need 50 to 100 billion CFUs (how we measure probiotic potency) with multiple strains of good bacteria to bring back the health of their microbiome.

RESET DETOX TIP #4: ELIMINATE TOXINS FROM YOUR
PLASTIC CONTAINERS

Your plastic bottles and food containers are filling you up with BPAs and phylates—remember those nasty endocrine disruptors we discussed in an earlier chapter? During your detox, only use BPA-free plastic bottles or change to glass bottles for your water. Make sure that your food containers at home are BPA-free or glass as well. And never microwave food in plastic containers (including plastic wrap, plastic bags, and plastic food storage containers like Tupperware). When you do, you cause the harmful chemicals in your plastics to leech out into your food and thus enter your body.

As a matter of fact, toss the microwave while you're at it. The process of microwaving food destroys all enzymes and vitamins in that food. It turns good food into dead food with no nutritional value. I have had many patients tell me that they microwave broccoli in a glass dish with plastic wrap over the top. Many people are eating broccoli for the health benefits, but when you microwave it with plastics, you kill the nutrients in it and harmful chemicals like phylates and BPAs leech into your food. The best way to cook your vegetables is to steam them on the stove.

RESET DETOX TIP #5: ELIMINATE TOXINS FROM YOUR HAIR
AND SKIN PRODUCTS

If you're like most women in the United States, you may put over five hundred chemicals on your skin every single day. Many of those chemicals, such as parabens, are known to cause cancer. Hard to believe? Well, it's true. A research study done by Bionsen, a natural deodorant company, found that the average woman's daily grooming and make-up routine causes her to "host" a staggering 515 different synthetic chemicals on her body every single day.[36] There are over 13,000 chemicals in cosmetics alone, and only 10 percent of them have been tested for safety.

---

36 Maureen Rice, "Revealed: The 515 Chemicals Women Put on Their Bodies Every Day," *Daily Mail*, updated November 20, 2009, http://www.dailymail.co.uk/femail/beauty/article-1229275/Revealed--515-chemicals-women-bodies-day.html.

Anything you put on your skin gets absorbed directly into your bloodstream and transported to the kidneys. What you put on your skin can destroy your health faster than what you put in your mouth. This includes lotions, makeup, shampoos, hairsprays, perfumes, soaps, etc.

Determining which products are harmful can be an overwhelming and confusing process. Use the Skin Deep app at http://www.ewg.org/skindeep/app/ to find out which products are safe and which ones are not safe.

My advice is that when you run out of a beauty product, replace it with a healthier option. Over time, you'll have only toxin-free products.

RESET DETOX TIP #6: ELIMINATE TOXIC HOUSEHOLD PRODUCTS

There are many toxins in the cleaning products you use in your home every single day. Most of them are way more toxic to your body than the food you consume. Start looking at your cleaners, detergents, air fresheners, and anything else that might be putting toxins in the air or touching your food. Check out the Environmental Working Group's healthy cleaning guide at http://www.ewg.org/guides/cleaners to learn more about which products you should avoid.

RESET DETOX TIP #7: FILTER YOUR WATER

Unfortunately, your water supply is another source from which you may be ingesting harmful chemicals. Investing in a reverse-osmosis water filter for drinking water is a smart idea. You can also have a water filter attached to your main water line so that all your faucets and spouts throughout your home will provide healthy water. If you're looking for the best option at the lowest price, Britta filters are also fantastic and a great option to start with.

When I first started learning about many of these toxins, avoiding them all felt like an impossible task. Then I realized that every step I took toward minimizing my exposure to them was a step in the right direction—and every little step counts. I've noticed that poor health and diseases can be really scary when you don't have a plan for getting and staying healthy. The purpose of this book is to educate you, empower you, and give you a rock-solid plan for lifelong health and vitality.

Follow the seven detox tips above for maximum results.

Overview of the 15-Day Detox

Here's an overview of what you'll do on a daily basis (you'll find details later in this chapter):

1. First thing in the morning upon rising, have a glass of Morning Detox water (see recipe chapter at the end of this book).

2. Replace two of your meals with detox smoothies. Make your first smoothie of the day for breakfast. Your second smoothie of the day can be either at lunch or at dinner—it's your choice.

3. Enjoy one meal per day with a clean protein, together with steamed vegetables or a fresh green salad.

4. Avoid all grains—including pasta, bread, cereal, rice, and corn.

5. Avoid all alcohol of any kind.

6. Avoid dairy of any kind—including cheese, milk, yogurt, and sour cream.

7. Enjoy five cups of raw vegetables a day; snacking on them throughout the day is encouraged.

8. Limit fruit to berries and green apples.

9. Any time you're feeling hungry during the day, you can eat all the green apples, berries, and vegetables you want.

10. For best results, take all supplements as directed on the protocol list (see "Supplements" section below).

WHAT YOU'LL NEED

Here's what you'll need to prepare for your 15-Day Detox program:

- *A blender.* My favorite is the Vitamix. You can get one easily at Costco, but any blender will do.
- *Plenty of fresh organic fruits and organic vegetables.* My favorites ones to munch on during the day are carrots, celery, red bell peppers, and green apples. My favorite ones to put into a smoothie are wild blueberries, cherries, and spinach. Keep in mind that you can always use frozen organic foods if fresh foods are not available.
- *A high-quality protein powder.* See the supplement list below for my recommendations.
- *Organic lemons* for your daily lemon water
- *Clean proteins*, like organic poultry, grass-fed beef, eggs from pasture-raised hens, hormone- and nitrite-free deli meats, and wild fish

- *Healthy and satisfying fats*, like avocados, coconut oil, and raw cashew and almond butters
- *Approved snacks*, such as raw nuts, red cabbage, hummus, kale chips, organic hard-boiled eggs, sweet potato chips, and non-GMO organic popcorn (see my favorite recipes in the back of the book)
- *Plenty of organic salad mixes and organic greens,* such as parsley, kale, romaine lettuce, and spinach
- *Supplements—those found on the list below*
- *A GREAT attitude!* You should be excited! You are about to experience what it's like to live in a body that is full of energy and that functions at a higher level than you may have ever experienced before.

YOUR DETOX SUPPLEMENTS

There is a wide range of quality in the supplement market, and many supplements do not provide the nutrition that the bottle promises. Often people reach for the cheapest supplement option, but the fact is that many of the supplements found at your local drugstore or grocery store are synthetic and can be toxic for your body. Therefore, during the 15-Day Detox, you will only consume high-quality food-based supplements that your body can instantly turn into nutrients. Here are the supplements with which I've had the best success in helping patients reset their health (amounts are recommended daily dosage):

➢ Probiotic (50 billion CFUs)
➢ Vitamin D3 (5,000 IU)
➢ Turmeric (225 mg)
➢ N Acetyl-L-Cysteine (100 mg)
➢ L-Glutamine (powder form) (5 g)
➢ Glutathione (250 mg)
➢ Milk Thistle (425mg)

➢ Alpha Lipoic Acid (ALA) (50mg)
➢ Plant-based or grass-fed whey protein powder (1 scoop)
➢ Greens superfood supplement with chlorophyll (1 scoop)
➢ Omega-3 fish oils (5 g)

I know that choosing supplements can be overwhelming. It can also be easy to dismiss using them on this detox—but don't. Your liver and gut need extra help. Not putting harmful foods into your body is a wonderful start, but the supplements help repair damage that has accumulated over the years. You want high-quality supplements that will give you results, not expensive urine in which all the vitamins get excreted from your body. If you need more guidance with supplements, check out www.resetfactor.com for a list of the supplements I use.

When you first take a high-powered probiotic like the one I'm recommending, you may notice temporary bloating in your abdomen, gas, or loose bowels. I have even had people break out in rashes. Those are all great signs, indicating die-off of bad bacteria. Stay the course. Those symptoms won't last long. On the other side of those symptoms will be a fabulous-feeling body.

YOUR MEAL REPLACEMENT SMOOTHIE

Your two smoothies a day will help to reset your metabolism and give your gut and liver a break. You want to use low-glycemic fruits such as berries in your smoothie to minimize sugar intake during the 15-Day Detox. Coconut milk or almond milk are both great liquid sources for the smoothies. Adding in healthy fats such as a tablespoon of coconut oil, half an avocado, or a tablespoon of raw almond or cashew butter is an excellent way to make sure your smoothie is satisfying. Then add in your protein powder, greens, and supplements.

Here are the ingredients for just one kind of great detox smoothie:

---

1 scoop protein powder
1 scoop green superfood supplement
1 scoop L-Glutamine
1 cup frozen organic berries
1 cup organic kale or spinach
1 tablespoon coconut oil
1 cup coconut milk or almond milk (organic, non-flavored, and no added sugar)
½ avocado
1 cup water

Avoid using the following in your smoothies:

> ➤ Fruit juice
> ➤ Yogurt
> ➤ Honey
> ➤ Coconut sugar
> ➤ Ice cream or frozen yogurt
> ➤ High-glycemic fruits like mango, papaya, pineapple, or banana

Look in the recipe section of this book for great smoothie ideas.

APPROVED MEAL INGREDIENTS

You'll enjoy one meal each day while on the 15-Day Detox. I have included lots of delicious, easy-to-prepare, and flavor-packed recipes in the back of the book for you to enjoy. Here's what you can eat:

- *Clean proteins,* like organic poultry, grass-fed beef, pasture-raised eggs, hormone- and nitrite-free deli meats, and wild fish
- *Plenty of fresh organic fruits and organic vegetables.* My favorite ones to munch on during the day are carrots, celery, red bell peppers, and green apples. My favorite ones to put into a smoothie are wild blueberries, blackberries, and spinach
- *Healthy and satisfying fats,* like avocados, coconut oil, and raw cashew and almond butters
- *Plenty of organic salad mixes and organic greens,* such as parsley, kale, romaine lettuce, and spinach
- *Probiotic rich foods and drinks,* such as kimchi, sauerkraut, tempeh, pickles, pickled fruits and vegetables, and raw kefir (only allowed raw with no added sugars)
- *Bone Broth,* which helps to heal and seal the gut. See recipes.

APPROVED DRINKS

- ➤ At least six to eight glasses of water every day
- ➤ Fresh-squeezed juice made with veggies and fruits from the "approved" list above (check out healing green drink in recipes)
- ➤ Kombucha tea
- ➤ Mineral water or club soda (without sugar)
- ➤ Herbal organic tea (green tea is a great detoxifier)
- ➤ Bone broth (see Appendix for recipe)

WHAT TO AVOID

- ➤ All *sugars,* such as sugar, honey, agave, maple syrup, and high-fructose corn syrup
- ➤ All *grains,* such as breads, pasta, quinoa, and rice
- ➤ All *fruits* (except berries and green apples)
- ➤ All *processed foods* (human-made food)
- ➤ All *coffee*
- ➤ All *alcohol*

WHAT A DETOX DAY LOOKS LIKE
UPON WAKING IN THE MORNING:

- ➤ Drink 1 glass of lemon water at room temperature.
- ➤ Take 1 probiotic (50 billion CFU).
- ➤ Take glutathione (250 mg).
- ➤ Take milk thistle (425mg).

BREAKFAST:

> ➤ One delicious and nutritious smoothie, which includes 1 scoop protein powder, 1 scoop greens, and 1 scoop L-glutamine (5 g)

AFTER MORNING SMOOTHIE:

> ➤ Take Acetyl-L-Cysteine 100 mg (2 tablets).
> ➤ Take Turmeric 225 mg (2 tablets).
> ➤ Take Vitamin D3 (5,000 IU).
> ➤ Take Omega-3 fish oils (3 g).

LUNCH:

> ➤ One delicious and nutritious smoothie, which includes 1 scoop protein powder, 1 scoop greens, and 1 scoop L-glutamine (5 g)

DINNER:

> ➤ One delicious and nutritious meal with clean protein, organic vegetables, and a fresh salad

SNACKS:

> ➤ Raw nuts, red cabbage, hummus, kale chips, organic hard-boiled eggs, green apples, and almond butter

BEFORE BED:

> ➤ Take 1 probiotic (50 billion CFU), preferably two hours after dinner.

WHAT TO EXPECT DAY BY DAY
DAYS 1 TO 3

No doubt, the first few days can be hard. You're helping your body begin to release toxins that have been stored for an extended period of time. In the first few days of this program, you can expect:

- Fatigue
- Headaches
- Increased bowel movements and urination
- Hunger

- Thirst
- Irritability
- Changes in mood
- Skin rashes or irritation

DAYS 4 TO 6

You're beginning to increase the amount of toxins you're releasing. You've started burning fat by changing the way you eat. You're extracting those toxins from your tissues and eliminating them by taking your supplements daily. Did you know that fat is where our body stores toxins?

Your cleanse is helping you to break down fat and finally rid your body of toxins.

The symptoms you experienced during days 1 to 3 can intensify during the next three days.

DAYS 7 TO 9

Depending on how toxic you are, by this point your symptoms should start improving. You're hitting the peak of your cleanse. The supplements, combined with your diet, are supporting the extraction and elimination of toxins. You may notice at this point that your stomach is flatter, your weight is dropping, and your energy is improving. If you're not experiencing those symptoms, don't worry. It means you just have more toxins to release. Stay the course and you'll soon feel the results.

DAYS 10 TO 12

You should now start to notice the benefits of your cleanse. If you've changed your diet, you'll notice that food is starting to taste better. At first, your new diet might have seemed bland, but now you're getting used to these new flavors.

Your body is acclimating to a new diet and improved nutrition, so you can expect the following:

- Improved energy
- Weight loss
- Improved sleep
- Improved digestion

DAYS 13 TO 15

By now you should be feeling great! You've eliminated a lot of the toxins you've previously accumulated over time. You might experience more of the same symptoms you felt during days 10 to 12.

The average weight loss with this detox is 8 pounds in 15 days. If you hit this point and you are not losing weight, then that can be an indication there are more toxins that need to be released. Don't be discouraged. As you move into your 30-Day Habit Reset, those toxins will continue to be released and your metabolism will gain momentum and speed up.

FREQUENTLY ASKED QUESTIONS
DO I HAVE TO DO TWO SMOOTHIES EVERY DAY?

Yes. The protein powder, superfood greens, and L-glutamine have specific nutrients that help the body in the detoxification process, so it's important to get two smoothies in per day. Some people prefer to have their one meal at lunch instead of dinner, and that's OK. Just make sure you're replacing two meals with the smoothies.

CAN I EAT MORE THAN ONE MEAL PER DAY?

It's recommended that you eat only one large meal. The timing of the meal is not important. If a smoothie is not filling enough and you feel like you need more food, feel free to eat approved snacks.

DO I HAVE TO TAKE THE VITAMINS WITH THE 15-DAY DETOX?

Yes. The vitamins are specifically selected to pull toxins from your body, repair your gut, lower any inflammation, stabilize your blood sugar, and cleanse your liver. Taking vitamins is extremely helpful to accelerating the detox process.

I'M A VEGETARIAN—CAN I STILL DO THE 15-DAY DETOX?

Of course! When using the protein powders, just be sure to use a plant, hemp, or pea protein. There are a lot of great sources of vegetarian protein powder out there. When it comes to your meal, do a vegetarian meal. Just avoid the clean protein. The mistake I often see vegetarians make is to eat a meal too high in carbohydrates, especially grain, pastas, and rice. Since the entire 45-Day Reset is about lowering your carbohydrates, be sure you don't add any high-carbohydrate grains or pastas to your daily routine.

I DIDN'T DO ALL THE TESTS YOU MENTION IN THIS BOOK. CAN I STILL DO THE 15-DAY DETOX?

Although it's advised that you be under a doctor's care while making any big changes to your diet, you don't need to have all the tests I do in my office to be successful at this program. This program will work with or without the testing. The tests I do, such as the organic acids test, helps me zero in on what the patient needs the most.

HELP! I'M HUNGRY!

If you find yourself starving, you need to eat more fat. Eat more avocados, raw nuts, or hummus. Make sure to add coconut oil to your smoothies. I even recommend taking a scoop of raw almond butter or raw cashew butter and eating it directly off your spoon. This is also a great tip if you crave sugar at night.

Also, make sure that you're not putting high-sugar fruits in your smoothies. Tropical fruits—such as pineapple, mango, and banana—are highest in sugar. These fruits will spike your blood sugar quickly and leave you feeling hungrier.

When I first rolled out this detox with my patients, it was after the holidays. People were complaining of how they had overindulged and needed to reset after all the toxins they had built up in December. The results were fantastic. The majority of people said their sugar and alcohol cravings went away quickly. Most said they weren't hungry. Some had a hard time the first few days with low energy, rashes, and foggy brain.

But by the end of the 15 days, everyone felt fantastic and *everyone* lost weight.

I then had people follow it up with the 30-Day Habit Reset. Once again, the results were incredible. Since toxins cause your body to hold onto weight, when people focused on pulling toxins out first, their weight loss in the 30-Day Reset was remarkable. People lost more weight than in any other 30-day program I have ever prescribed.

The amazing piece was that even months later, people had kept the weight off and were still feeling great. Even if they cheated a little here and there, they had truly reset their health. Years later, I have done this 45-Day Reset with thousands of people—all with the same result. This program works. And it will give you permanent results.

So hang in there through the tough days—your body will thank you. Remember that two of the keys to healing are time and repetition. Every day you're on this program, you'll build your body stronger and stronger. Eventually, momentum and healing take over, and cravings and hunger go away. It's at this moment that I see a magical look in people's eyes. It's a look of deep satisfaction—a feeling of self-pride. There is no greater feeling than knowing you are in control of your own health. You get to decide how you feel and what direction your health will head. Nothing tastes as good as that!

Now on to your 30-day Habit Reset, where you'll learn how to teach your body to crave health more than any dessert placed in front of you.

CHAPTER 11

The 30-Day Habit Reset

CONGRATULATIONS! THE HARDEST PART IS over. Now that you've completed your 15-Day GI and Liver Detox, move immediately into your 30-Day Habit Reset. The great news is that you get to eat more meals, drink fewer smoothies (if you want), and have all the fruit you want.

I'm often asked "Can I keep doing the smoothies? I feel great and enjoy them." My answer is YES! You don't have to stop the smoothies or vitamins if you're feeling good—that part is optional as we move into the 30-Day Habit Reset.

The 30-Day Habit Reset is designed to help you create lasting good health habits that you can easily stick to for life. There's no break in between the 15-Day GI and Liver Reset and the 30-Day Habit Reset. This is meant to be a 45-day program that you follow straight through.

WHAT TO DO DURING YOUR 30-DAY HABIT RESET:

- Continue to follow the 8 Reset Rules of Health (see Chapter 8).
- Continue to stay off all grains, pastas, and white potatoes.
- Continue to stay off all alcohol.
- Continue to stay off sugar.
- Continue to stay off bad fats and processed foods.
- Continue to eat as many raw organic vegetables as you possibly can throughout the day.

- You can add back in more meals. Eat as many meals as you want (you don't have to stick to only one meal).
- You can add back in raw organic cow dairy, goat dairy, or sheep dairy. Still

stay away from pasteurized conventional dairy.
- You can add back in ALL organic fruits.
- The only GI supplements required are probiotic, L-glutamine, and omega-3s.

RULES FOR THE 30-DAY HABIT RESET

Remember, the 30-day part of the 45-Day Reset is designed to help you change your health habits *as a lifestyle*. We've talked about many of these already, but here's an important overview of the effects of sugar, alcohol, grains, dairy, etc., and how to create new and positive habits around these substances.

RESET RULES OF SUGAR

You may feel nervous about continuing to avoid sugar during the 30-day Habit Reset, but let me tell you, there are great alternatives to refined white sugar. Over the next 30 days, you can have as much stevia and xylitol as you desire. You may also add coconut sugar, but do so in moderation. You'll notice the recipes in the back of the book include these sugars.

My experience has been that not everyone likes stevia; many people prefer coconut sugar. If you're looking at a new recipe and it calls for sugar, coconut sugar has a 1–1 ratio to refined sugar. If the recipe calls for a cup of sugar, replace it with a cup of coconut sugar.

A question I'm asked frequently is "What about organic refined sugar?" Remember that the 45-Day Reset is designed to kick your body out of an insulin-resistant state; unfortunately, even organic refined sugar will cause your pancreas to work too hard and keep your insulin receptor sites blocked. See Chapter 9 for the list of hidden names for sugars. Avoid all of them to make sure you get the best results.

RESET RULES OF OIL

As I mentioned in earlier chapters, the United States is one of the most fat-deprived nations. You absolutely need fat to keep your body healthy. So for the next 30 days, you're going to substitute good, health-promoting fats for all bad, harmful, inflammatory fats.

Eliminate inflammatory fats such as:

- Canola oil
- Safflower oil
- Sunflower oil
- Vegetable oil
- Crisco
- Margarine

Substitute bad fats with these health-promoting fats:

- Avocado oil
- Olive oil (don't heat above 100 degrees)
- Coconut oil
- Sesame oil
- Grapeseed oil
- Organic butter (from pasture-raised cows' milk)

RESET RULES OF DAIRY

The pasteurization process causes dairy to have a higher sugar content, so when you buy dairy, always look for raw dairy. This is usually pretty easy when you're searching for cheese but a lot more difficult when you're looking for milk. You'll notice in the 15-Day GI and Liver Detox that you're not to eat any dairy. This is because I want to take out of your diet any food that could harm your gut or cause you to be insulin resistant. Read Chapter 2, "Your Gut Instincts Are Right," to learn more about this harmful food.

Many people are sensitive to dairy, so as you add dairy back into your diet after the 15-Day Detox, it needs to be raw organic dairy and you need to notice if you have any kind of reaction after eating it. A reaction to dairy might be bloating, skin rash, or overall feelings of sluggishness.

Research has found that a glass of milk can contain a cocktail of twenty painkillers, antibiotics, and growth hormones. It also contains estrogen-mimicking hormones—as we discussed in the "Your Gut Instincts Are Right" and "Calories Don't Count-Hormones Do" chapters—leading to breast cancer and other hormonal imbalances. The other challenge with cow's milk is that the size of cow's milk molecules is significantly bigger than that of human breast milk molecules. Our bodies were designed to break down human breast milk, not these larger milk molecules. Goat's milk is a great alternative, as it contains smaller molecules that are easier for our digestive system to handle.

RESET RULES OF EGGS

You can eat as many eggs as you want during both your 15-Day GI and Liver Detox and your 30-Day Habit Reset. When buying eggs, make sure you get organic, cage-free eggs. Those are going to have the most nutrients with the least number of harmful chemicals. Pasture-raised organic eggs are the absolute best, and you'll notice that their yoke color is a deep orange/yellow. They are filled with more helpful nutrients, and fewer harmful alterations have been made to the chickens that lay them.

RESET RULES OF GRAINS

Grains turn to sugar once they enter the bloodstream. A piece of bread is said to have as high a glycemic index as a candy bar.[37] Like

---

37 "Glycemic Index and Glycemic Load for 100+ Foods," Harvard Health Publications website, February 3, 2015, http://www.health.harvard.edu/healthy-eating/glycemic_index_and_glycemic_load_for_100_foods/

consuming sugar, consuming grains is one of the fastest paths to gaining weight. This is one of the reasons I have you continue to remove grains from your diet during the 30-Day Habit Reset. Although I like gluten-free flours, which are better for your gut than wheat and white bread, for the whole 45 days I want you to pull out ALL grains. This is the fastest path to weight loss and health. However, that doesn't mean you'll never be able to have your muffins, pancakes, and breads again; there are great alternatives to wheat and white flour.

Here's a list of foods that you should avoid during your 30-Day Habit Reset program:

- White bread (use Paleo Bread instead)
- All pastas (use zucchini noodles and sweet potato noodles instead)
- White and red potatoes (use sweet potatoes instead)
- Rye bread
- Whole wheat bread
- Muffins (substitute almond and coconut flour in a recipe)
- English muffins
- Baked goods and pastries
- Crackers
- Potato chips
- Pie crust
- Cookies
- Brown and white rice (use wild rice and quinoa instead)
- Corn and corn chips
- Popcorn
- Corn and flour tortillas (use Paleo Wraps instead)

Avoid these flours if you see them listed on a label, as they're high in sugar:

- White flour
- Whole wheat flour
- Sourdough flour
- Rye flour
- Barley flour
- Graham flour
- Matzo flour
- Malt flour
- Durum flour
- Couscous flour
- Bulgur flour
- Semolina flour
- Brown rice flour
- Spelt flour
- Kamut flour
- Amaranth flour
- Arrowroot flour
- Buckwheat flour
- Corn flour
- Corn meal
- Millet flour
- Oat flour
- Potato flour
- Quinoa flour
- Sorghum flour
- Tapioca flour
- Teff flour
- White rice flour

Other starches to avoid:

- White rice
- Brown rice
- White potatoes
- Oats

Here are great approved substitutions that you can eat:

- Paleo Wraps (substitute for tortillas) (Check out Thrive Market online.)

Flour substitutes with low sugar include the following (you can have these on the 30-Day Habit Reset):

- Almond flour
- Coconut flour
- Hemp flour
- Lupin flour
- Chickpea flour
- Chia flour

RESET RULES OF FRUITS AND VEGETABLES

First, eat only organic fruits and vegetables. Second, keep vegetables raw since raw vegetables are more beneficial to your body than cooked vegetables. Once you cook vegetables, you destroy many of their nutrients. Make a point of having raw vegetables at every meal. The only exception to this is if you feel bloated after you eat. People who have too much bad bacteria, as with SIBO, can feel extremely bloated after eating raw vegetables. If this is your experience, cut back on the raw vegetables and give your gut more time to repair. Keep trying to add raw vegetables back in every few days. If you are taking a high-powered probiotic, with enough time, the bloated feeling will go away and you'll be able to eat more raw vegetables.

The other thing to think about with fruits and vegetables is their sugar content. Many people are surprised to hear that these healthy foods have a high sugar content, but they can as easily raise your blood sugar as organic refined sugar can.

Highest-sugared vegetables—eat only in moderation:

- Carrots
- Beets

Medium-sugared vegetables—eat as much as you want:

- Red, yellow, and orange peppers
- Red cabbage
- Tomatoes

Lowest-sugared vegetables—eat as much as you want:

- Green lettuces
- Parsley
- Celery

- Avocados
- Cucumber
- Kale
- Green cabbage
- Cauliflower

Highest-sugared fruits—avoid during your entire 45-Day Reset:

- Tropical fruits such as pineapple, papaya, mango, banana, and grapes.

Medium-sugared fruits—avoid during your 15-Day Detox, but eat in moderation during your 30-Day Habit Reset:

- Citrus fruits
- Melons
- Nectarines
- Peaches
- Pears
- Apples (except green)
- Kiwi

Lowest-sugared fruits—eat as much as you want throughout your entire 45-Day Reset:

- Any kind of berries—including strawberries, rasp-berries, blueberries, blackberries, boysenberries, huckleberries
- Green apples

When it comes to deciding whether to buy your fruits and vegetables organic, I recommend that you try to buy as many organics as possible. If money is a consideration, we've talked about the EWG's Dirty Dozen and Clean Fifteen lists. The Dirty Dozen are those fruits and vegetable most heavily sprayed with pesticides. You want to buy these organic. The Clean Fifteen, on the other hand, are not as heavily sprayed with pesticides; it's safer to eat conventional versions of these, if you have to. Here are the lists for easy reference:

The Clean Fifteen (OK to buy nonorganic):

- Onions
- Avocados
- Pineapple
- Mangoes
- Sweet peas
- Eggplant
- Cauliflower
- Asparagus
- Kiwi
- Cabbage
- Watermelon
- Grapefruit
- Sweet Potatoes
- Honeydew Melon

You may have noticed that this list contains only 14 fruits and vegetables. I removed sweet corn from the list because corn is one of the most genetically modified crops and should *only* be bought organic.

The Dirty Dozen (always buy organic):

- Apples
- Celery
- Tomatoes
- Cucumber
- Grapes
- Nectarines
- Peaches
- Potatoes
- Spinach
- Strawberries
- Blueberries
- Sweet bell peppers

Some experts suggest that you add kale and green beans to this list, as these have been more heavily sprayed in recent years. I also would add corn to this list due to the fact that it is genetically modified.

RESET RULES OF MEAT AND FISH

Unfortunately, if you're eating grain-fed beef, you're getting a large dose of antibiotic and hormone-injected meat. Every chemical that's put into the animal, including the chemical-laden food that animal is fed, is still in the meat as it sits on your dinner plate. These chemicals slow down your digestion, making you bloated or constipated, and they raise your estrogen levels. Grain-fed meat also typically has more fat than other meats. Toxins live in the fat of an animal. When you eat that fat, you're getting all those toxins the liver tried to excrete and ended up storing in the fat.

According to Dr. Sara Gottfried in her book *The Hormone Reset Diet*, we are hardwired by our DNA and the microbes in our gut to eat mostly vegetables, nuts, seeds, occasional fruit, and clean protein. Eating this way will keep you lean and your hormones balanced.

During your 45-Day Reset, you can have organic meat and fish in moderation. Since meat carries the highest amount of toxins, it's imperative that you go organic. If money is a concern, I would rather you bought your meats organic and your fruits and vegetables nonorganic. Just be sure to follow the guidelines set out by the EWG when buying foods from the Dirty Dozen and Clean Fifteen lists.

Here's what else you need to know about various meats:

- **Beef:** Avoid all grain-fed beef. A great alternative to grain-fed beef is grass-fed beef. Unlike grain-fed beef, grass-fed beef is incredibly good for your body. Beef from cows that are allowed to graze on grass and roam in large fields is high in omega-3 oils that are crucial for improving brain function, lowering inflammation, and keeping your metabolism working efficiently. Include grass-fed beef in your meals at least twice a week.
- **Chicken:** Organic chicken of all types (drumsticks, wings, breasts, skin-on) is OK. Nonorganic chicken is packed with antibiotics and hormones that have been injected into the animals. Avoid nonorganic chicken at all costs.
- **Fish:** Farm-fresh fish is an absolute no-no, as it lacks key nutrients like omega-3 oils. Frozen or fresh fish is fine, but all fish should be wild, not farm raised. Sometimes you have to ask your butcher or waiter at a restaurant if the fish is wild.

Here's the Food & Water Watch's "dirty dozen" list of seafood. Avoid these during your 45-Day Reset:

- King crab
- Caviar
- Atlantic bluefin tuna
- Orange roughy
- Atlantic flatfish
- American eel
- American cod
- Imported catfish
- Chilean seabass
- Shark
- Atlantic and farmed salmon
- Imported shrimp
- Tilapia

Deli Meats: These meats carry the highest possibility of toxic overload, so you absolutely want these meats organic and nitrite-free. Several studies have been done on the increase in incidents of leukemia in kids who eat processed deli meats. Sausages, salamis, and sliced turkey are all great choices when bought organic and free from nitrites.

Pork: This is the one meat you want to eat in moderation or cut out completely. The pig is the only animal that does not have sweat glands and thus holds on to all of its toxins. Since the 45-Day Reset is about detoxifying your body, I highly recommend you eat pork rarely or not at all. If you do choose to eat pork, be sure that it's organic and has no caramel coloring or sodium nitrites in it.

RESET RULES OF ALCOHOL

Next to pulling grains out of your diet, this is everyone's least favorite nutritional habit. Yet pulling alcohol out of your diet will have a significant effect on your overall health. During your 45-Day Reset, you are to pull ALL alcohol out of your diet.

Many people love a glass of wine at night after a hard day at work. So I'm sorry to be the bearer of bad news: even one glass raises your estrogen levels, kills good bacteria in your gut, and stops your liver from metabolizing fat for energy. If you're trying to reset your health, drinking alcohol will hold you back from living in the body you deserve to live in.

Recently, a family member of mine wanted some weight loss advice. She'd been thin most her life but was noticing that she was starting to hold on to weight more than ever. She had been eating and drinking the same way for years and was surprised as the number on her scale started getting higher and higher.

She got motivated and joined a gym. She made a new health habit of daily workouts, hoping this would cause her to lose weight. After weeks of committing to her new exercise regime, she hadn't lost a single pound. She was frustrated and ready to give up on her workout plan. When I sat down with her to look at her diet, I could see that she ate fairly well. The problem was that she loved drinking beer. And while she was practicing many of the right health habits to be the weight she wanted, the beer had caught up with her.

What happens when you drink alcohol? Several chemical processes happen that don't benefit you. First, you destroy your gut. Beer and wine have the highest amount of yeast in them. One of the major breakdowns of the gastrointestinal system is candida. Drinks like beer and wine feed candida, causing you to crave more beer and wine. A great way to stop the cravings is to stop feeding your body yeast. It can be difficult at first, but as the candida dies over time, so will your cravings.

Second, alcohol increases estrogen in your body. Now, remember that estrogen is what makes a female body curvy. The more estrogen you have in your system, the more your body will convert that to fat. Even one glass of alcohol per day can make you put on extra pounds. During your 45-Day Reset, you're going to pull all alcohol from your diet. For some of you, this may be hard, but I promise if you hang in there and give it enough time, you'll see the benefits quickly as the fat around your abdomen starts to disappear.

Third, as long as your liver is metabolizing the alcohol, it can't burn fat. Many studies have shown how alcohol causes the body to stop the burning of fat for energy. For some of you, this is going to be the hardest part of your reset experience. But the whole idea of the 45-Day Reset is to bring your body back to its original state, the way it was designed to be. You can't fully reset without giving up alcohol. Give your liver a break and watch your body flourish!

Although you won't be drinking alcohol during your 45-Day Reset, once your reset is over, drinking alcohol in moderation (1 to 2 drinks a week) is not harmful. But you do need to know a few key things about alcohol and how it's processed in the body.

- **Beer:** This is probably the worst alcoholic beverage you can drink because of its high gluten and yeast content. Hopefully, if you've made it this far in the book, you know by now that the key to living with lifelong health starts by taking good care of your gut. Beer will quickly destroy the good bacteria in your gut and increase your estrogen levels, leaving you bloated and hanging on to extra fat. Sound appealing? I would avoid beer at all costs.

- **Wine:** Although there are many scientific papers showing that the high antioxidant content of wine is beneficial to the body, the sulfites and high sugar content in wine are both destructive to the gut and stressful to the pancreas. If you remember the "Resetting Your Gut" chapter, many people suffer from candida. Candida is caused by too much yeast—and most wines are packed with yeast. Bottom line: wine has too much sugar in it, and whenever you're trying to keep your weight down, avoiding wine is a good practice.

> • **Mixed Drinks:** The biggest challenge with mixed drinks is what you mix the alcohol with. Since we're trying to minimize your sugar content, mixing your gin with tonic gives you a burst of sugar that could easily put you back into insulin resistance. Hard liquor has less sugar than many nonalcoholic drinks, and if it's mixed with something mellow, such as a club soda, it's your best choice of alcoholic beverage.

RESET RULES OF NONALCOHOLIC DRINKS

The bottom line here is that you want to drink water—and lots of it! If you're fine for the next 45 days drinking *only* water, that is the quickest path to success! Other great choices for nonalcoholic drinks are herbal teas, kombucha, club soda, zevias, or green juices with limited fruit.

Coffee drinking is not recommended during your 45-Day Reset. When drinking coffee *after* your 45 days, make sure it's organic, as many coffees have fungus on them and are heavily sprayed. If you have an extreme coffee habit, you'll want to slowly limit your coffee during your reset period to minimize headaches and extreme fatigue.

The best way to get off coffee is to have a little less each day. If you serve yourself a quarter of a cup less every day, over a few days to a week you'll be completely off it without any headaches or extreme exhaustion. The other thing about coffee that destroys people's health is what they put in their coffee. Added sugar, nonorganic dairy, artificial sweeteners, creamers, syrups, and whipped cream are all destroyers of your health.

Organic herbal teas are a great alternative to coffee. Green tea and yerba mate tea will give you an energy lift without draining your adrenal glands like coffee does.

RESET RULES OF HOW OFTEN AND HOW MUCH TO EAT

The 45-Day Reset is not a food deprivation plan. You can eat as much as you want of the approved foods at whatever time you want to eat. The only time of the day I highly recommend limiting your food intake is before bed. The reason for this is that going to bed with a full stomach often causes food to ferment in your gut, which can destroy good bacteria and increase your chances of candida. Also, your body cannot properly digest and metabolize food that you eat right before bed. In fact, as mentioned earlier, one of the strategies sumo wrestlers use to fatten up is to always take a nap after their largest meal. Going to sleep on a full stomach forces the body to store most of the calories as fat, as it doesn't have the ability to metabolize large amounts of food while sleeping.

Studies used to show that you needed three meals a day and that you needed to eat first thing in the morning. This is an outdated theory; eat when you want to eat. As your body resets and comes back to its original design, it will tell you when it's hungry. Honor that. A well-functioning body knows best.

RESET RULES FOR EATING OUT

While you're doing your 15-Day GI and Liver Detox, it may be difficult to eat out. During the 30-Day Habit Reset, eating out should be a little easier. The one major challenge you'll find with eating out is that you won't have control over the quality of the food you eat. Most restaurants use nonorganic GMO food. They also tend to cook with the wrong oils. Because of this, eating out on a regular basis can be a fast path to poor health and packing on the pounds. Many studies have found that people eating in a restaurant eat 40 percent more food and 30 percent more bad fat than they would if they were at home.

When you do eat out, there are some smart guidelines you can follow. When ordering from a menu, go directly to the salad section or the entrée section. Hors-d'oeuvres and desserts are most likely to be non-approved foods. Eating out often during your 30-Day Habit Reset is not advised, but if an invitation arises, don't feel as if you can't participate. Other tips: when the waiter brings the bread, tell him or her not to leave it on the table. Many people find it hard not to munch on the bread, so if it's out of your sight, it'll be easier to avoid! The other item people find difficult is drinks; stick with water or tea.

RESET RULES FOR GROCERY SHOPPING

I highly recommend looking through the recipes in the back of this book and picking out some key recipes you want to make. Make a list of exactly what you're going to purchase. Realize that most processed foods and foods that will destroy your health are located in the center aisles of the grocery store. The fresh food is around the edges, so stick to the vegetable, meat, eggs, and refrigerated foods sections; that's where the healthiest food lives.

I also recommend that you never go to the grocery store hungry, as bad decisions usually result. Also, if you have a well-organized list, you won't be distracted by foods that you normally wouldn't have bought prior to your 45-Day Reset.

MENU IDEAS

Sometimes patients will tell me that they understand the concepts I've described in this book but are not quite sure how to put them into action. This is why I have put recipes in the back to help give you some good ideas. Many of these recipes are ones that I use on a daily basis with my family. But to give you a better idea of meal planning, the following are examples of foods that I recommend for each meal.

BREAKFAST

- Smoothies
- Breakfast salad (fried eggs on top of greens)
- Egg and avocado
- Hard-boiled or soft-boiled eggs

The keys to a healthy breakfast are protein and fats. Eating these at the start of the day will minimize your hunger and give you sustained energy throughout your morning. But what many people reach for at breakfast is a pastry or cereal. There is too much sugar in both those options, which is why many people get hungry at ten o'clock and start craving something sugary or caffeinated to lift up their energy.

LUNCH

Again, the strategy at lunch is controlling your blood sugar. Protein, vegetables, and healthy fats are the best things you can have for lunch. If you notice a three o'clock dip, what you ate for lunch spiked your blood sugar too high. When your blood sugar spikes at high noon, it will crash at 3:00 p.m. and have you craving something sugary. This is very similar to the 10:00 a.m. dip some people feel.

Most people don't experience these dips on their 45-Day Reset because the program is geared toward controlling your blood sugar. But if you ever experience extreme hunger and low energy, remember the key is to decrease your sugar (usually from fruit or too much protein) and increase your fat (with more avocado, raw nuts, raw nut butter, and hummus).

The following are good lunch ideas:

- Salad with clean protein (see salad section)
- A grainless sandwich
- Clean protein with cooked vegetables

DINNER

This is the most important meal of the day. What you eat at dinner will determine how much insulin will be floating in your bloodstream while you sleep. If you're waking up exhausted, then you're eating too many things that increase the release of insulin. These are the same things that cause your energy to crash at 10:00 a.m. and 3:00 p.m.

One of the mistakes I see people make on the 30-Day Habit Reset is eating too many fruits or too much protein. If you're waking up exhausted or not losing as much weight as you would like on this program, look at what you're eating at dinner. Less protein, fewer fruits, and more fats and vegetables are the key to balancing your insulin levels and speeding up your metabolism.

The following are some of my recommendations for dinner:

- Roasted chicken with cooked vegetables and sweet potatoes
- Grass-fed burgers wrapped in butter lettuce with avocado and sweet potato coins
- Wild-caught salmon with sautéed bok choy
- Fish tacos with Paleo wraps

LATERAL CHANGES

In this 45-Day Reset, you'll see that I like to incorporate a lot of "lateral" changes. What I mean by *lateral changes* is that you're going to just swap out a food you're already eating for a healthier choice. Switching from grain-fed beef to grass-fed beef is a great example of that. When you go to the market, just commit to only buying grass-fed beef.

In the beginning, it will taste different. The first time I tasted grass-fed beef years ago, I was unsure that I could grow to like it. But with time and repetition, you'll notice that the taste becomes what you're used to. Remember that you've trained yourself to like the foods you eat now. If those foods are not building you a healthy body, make some lateral changes. Know that the new taste will be different at first—but don't let that stop you. Stay with it. Grass-fed beef has so much to offer you and your health!

If you're missing some of your favorite foods, ask yourself if there's a good lateral change you can make that might be a healthier choice. Here are some of the more common lateral changes I recommend:

- Coconut sugar for refined sugar
- Zevia sodas for regular sodas
- Coconut oil for canola oil
- Raw nuts for roasted nuts
- Paleo wraps for tortillas
- Romaine lettuce for bread (I know it's not the same, but it works!)
- Grainless bread for regular bread
- Sweet potatoes for white potatoes
- Nitrite-free deli meats for processed meats
- Wild salmon for farm-raised salmon
- Grass-fed beef for grain-fed beef
- Lily's chocolates for processed candy
- Kombucha for beer

These are just a few examples that have worked for many of my patients. Your first reaction may be that the lateral change is nowhere near the original food. Remember that you have trained your taste buds to love these foods—so you can train them differently. It takes time and repetition of the new foods for your brain and taste buds to like them. But give it a shot. Be adventurous. The more you add these great new healthy foods into your diet, the more normal they will feel.

INTERMITTENT FASTING

This concept is an advanced nutritional idea. It's advanced because for many of you who will be getting off sugar and grains, it will be a huge change. And fasting may be the furthest thing from your mind. But I want to include fasting in this book because it's getting so much attention as a fantastic way to slow down the aging process, stop insulin resistance, and reverse diseases like cancer.

According to Dr. Daniel Pompa, author of *The Cellular Healing Diet*, fasting markedly improves almost every health condition. It does this by down-regulating cellular inflammation. Since inflammation has been named the silent killer—linked to almost every chronic disease, including cancer—lowering cellular inflammation is a powerful step in resetting your body. There is no faster way to lower inflammation than to fast.

A recent study suggested that fasting for three consecutive days actually "flips a switch" to ignite regeneration of the immune system.[38] It's the ultimate reset button, actually triggering the body to begin producing new white blood cells. The study also found that prolonged fasting triggered a reduction of the enzyme PKA, which is linked to aging and increased risk of cancer and tumor growth. According to scientists at the University of Southern California, "There is no evidence at all

---

38   Sarah Knapton, "Fasting for Three Days Can Regenerate Entire Immune System, Study Finds," *The Telegraph*, June 5, 2014, http://www.telegraph.co.uk/news/uknews/10878625/Fasting-for-three-days-can-regenerate-entire-immune-system-study-finds.html.

that fasting would be dangerous while there is strong evidence that it is beneficial."[39]

If you're not convinced yet, fasting also spikes your growth hormone. If you remember from the "Resetting Your Hormones" chapter, growth hormone burns fat and slows the aging process. Fasting is also said to boost your energy because your body is not wasting energy on digesting food. This also helps take the burden off your gut when it needs to heal. Conditions like leaky gut, irritable bowel syndrome, and Crohn's Disease have all shown signs of improvement when a person fasted.

Other benefits of fasting include these:

- Weight loss
- Increased brain function and cognitive skills
- Powerful detoxification effects
- Life extension
- Improved hormone balance
- Insulin sensitivity
- Enhanced digestion
- Decreased disease risk
- Reduced appetite
- Improved immune function

Convinced yet?

So what's the best way to fast? Intermittent fasting is a fantastic way to fast without missing out completely on food. You'll want to go 15 to 18 hours without food. That means you'll be eating most of your food within a six- to nine-hour window.

This is how it works. Stop eating at 8:00 p.m. When you wake up in the morning, have some green tea with grass-fed raw cream or grass-fed organic butter in it. The saturated fats will help wake your brain up. After the 15-Day Detox, you can do organic coffee with grass-fed raw dairy.

Eat your first meal around noon. That would be sixteen hours without food (you can go longer if you want). Your first meal will be a light lunch with lots of healthy fats. Between five and eight hours from this

39 Ibid.

meal, you can eat however much you want. But this will be your biggest meal of the day.

Since you'll be eating less food overall, you'll need to make sure every calorie counts. Your dinner will need to be packed with protein and healthy fats. If you don't get a well-balanced dinner, you may have trouble sleeping and wake up hungry. Intermittent fasting, when done correctly, will stabilize your blood sugar to the point that hunger is a thing of the past.

If you want to try this type of fasting, I recommend you do it after your 15-Day Detox, when your blood sugar has already evened out and your brain is used to less food.

What About Exercise?

There's no doubt that our bodies were made to move. So during your 45-Day Reset, I highly recommend that you move your body every day. Since everyone starting this program is at a different starting point, the general formula I recommend is 3 days of walking per week, 20 minutes at a time; 3 days of Surge Training (see description below); and 1 day of yoga or stretching per week.

I have found over the years that your brain will start to negotiate with you if you only work out two to three times a week. Your brain will tell you "Oh, I'll do it tomorrow," and it will be easy to keep putting off. But if you know you have to move your body every day, it's just a matter of picking what type of movement you want to do—and the negotiating stops.

Research is also showing us that strenuous exercise, such as half-marathons or long triathlons, can be damaging to the heart and raise your cortisol levels. So for most people I don't recommend these types of activities unless it's their passion and they're training like extreme athletes.

Your exercise program has to have a good balance of cardiovascular training, weight training, and stretching. Many people, when they want to lose weight, want to hop on the treadmill for hours at a time. But as I mentioned before, this will raise your cortisol levels. When your cortisol goes up, your blood sugar goes down, and when your blood sugar goes down, you become more hungry and hold on to more fat. So for most people who are trying to lose weight, I don't recommend long periods of cardiovascular exercise.

On the other hand, when you start doing strength training and increase your muscle mass, it increases your metabolism. In fact, did you know that while you're sitting at your desk all day, you burn more calories if you have more muscle? Don't be scared to add some strength training to your weekly workout regime. There are many great "boot camps" around the country designed to do exactly this. Or meet with a personal trainer at your gym to get on a strength training program. It will benefit you greatly.

Example of Surge Training

If you don't have access to a gym or boot camp, here is an example of a Surge protocol that I teach at my office. Pick five of your favorite exercises. You can pick anything—if you don't like jumping jacks, pick a different exercise. The important thing is that when you do the exercises, you're able to do them without hurting yourself. Since Surging is about getting your heart rate up and down, try to push yourself until you're out of breath. Also check out my website at Resetfactor.com for more details.

Five Exercises:
  Jumping jacks
  Push-ups
  Running in place
  Running with high knees
  Tricep dips

INSTRUCTIONS:
One round of this surge protocol consists of ten steps:

1. Warm up for 1 minute by running in place.
2. Do jumping jacks as fast as you can for 30 seconds. Rest for 30 seconds.
3. Do push-ups as fast as you can for 30 seconds.
4. Rest for 30 seconds.
5. Run in place for 30 seconds.
6. Rest for 30 seconds.
7. Run in place with high knees for 30 seconds.
8. Rest for 30 seconds.
9. Do tricep dips for 30 seconds.
10. Rest for 30 seconds.

Repeat for a total of three rounds.

And that's it! What you do when you bring your heart rate up and down is train your body to speed up its metabolism and secrete growth hormone. If you remember from the "Resetting Your Hormone" chapter, growth hormone makes you burn fat and slows the aging process.

WHAT TO DO WHEN YOUR 45 DAYS IS OVER

When most people get to the end of their 45-Day Reset, they feel and look so good that they don't want to go back to their old habits. If this is you, I would encourage you to do the same. The reset rules I have outlined in this chapter are how I eat most the time—but I have what I call an 80/20 rule. Unless you're trying to reverse a disease or lose weight, 80 percent of the time, stick to the reset rules and everything you learned during your 45-Day Reset. The other 20 percent of the time, eat however you want. If you follow that formula, you most likely will avoid disease.

Now, if you get to the end of the 45 days and haven't lost as much weight as you wanted, or if you aren't feeling better, you need to follow the 90/10 rule: 90 percent of the time, you'll follow the reset rules, and 10 percent of the time, you can eat however you want. Ten percent equates to about two meals a week. Keep going, though. Don't be discouraged. I've seen some people need more time than 45 days to reset their health. It took you years to get to this place with your health; it can take some time to reverse it.

If you're trying to reverse disease, such as cancer, I strongly urge you to follow this nutrition program 100 percent of the time until your health is balanced and in a great place. Reversing disease takes serious commitment and can't be done moderately. You need to be all in! Many of my patients who have cancer or autoimmune conditions follow the Reset Program for years.

Remember, the key to success with any nutrition program is consistency. The first month, you'll see and feel your body changing; the second month, your friends and family will notice the changes; and by the third month, the *whole world* will begin to notice!

Conclusion

HOPEFULLY BY NOW, YOU KNOW that it is possible to reset your health. It doesn't matter how poor your lifestyle has been up to this point, how many times you've tried to get your health on track and failed, what your family history says about the diseases you're likely to get, or even what the diagnosis presently staring you in the face is. *Your body is built to heal!*

There are two ways to approach your health. One is with the attitude that you have no control; the other is that you have ALL the control. I preach the second approach. I've watched too many people succeed at changing the direction of their health to know that it's possible. I also know the path I've outlined for you in this book will give you back that control.

Be patient. Have faith. Surround yourself with people who believe in you. Don't ever take no for an answer. There is always a way to move your body toward health—you just have to keep taking action and keep applying the principles I've outlined for you here.

Every morning when you wake up, write down three steps you're going to take that day to build health. Keep your mind focused on those steps. Don't look back—you're not heading in that direction. It doesn't matter what you've done with your body up until now—you're on a new path now, one that has you living in the body you've always dreamed of.

If you slip, don't let it get you down. You can always hop back on your new program. You have within you the most powerful doctor that ever lived. Your body wants to heal. The more you follow the principles in this book, the stronger you make that doctor.

I have dedicated this book to a dear friend of mine who refused to take no for an answer. At 40, she was given a diagnosis of metastatic breast cancer. She had gone for a routine mammogram and had come away a cancer patient with a death sentence. She had had no warning signs and no symptoms, and she was sideswiped by this horrible diagnosis.

But she set out to defeat it at all odds. When the doctors told her she had months to live, she turned it into over a decade. When she was told chemotherapy and surgery were her only choices of treatment, she found a team of doctors who showed her several ways to build health and kill cancer naturally. When most people would be fearful and shut down, she developed a mindset of leaving no stone unturned in search of answers.

She did everything possible to find answers. She surrounded herself with people who believed in her and cheered her on. She kept herself in action every day and never gave up. She only focused on moving forward, never beating herself up for what she had done or hadn't done in the past. She had one mission: stay healthy and happy as long as possible.

No matter where you are today with your health, I want the same strategy for you. I want you to believe in yourself and see only solutions. Be patient. It may take you some time, but the principles in this book are proven to work. Stop searching for shortcuts— they don't exist when it comes to health. Changing your habits and committing to improving your health is a process.

Let go of fear. It's not serving you. There are only possibility and hope on the path to health. Believe in miracles. You *are* a miracle. Your body heals cancer cells every day. While you've been reading this book, thousands—if not millions—of people have been reversing their disease. The last chapters of your life haven't been written yet; you get to write them now. You get to set your health in the direction YOU choose.

I'll end with this thought: if disease builds in your body from poor lifestyle habits practiced over and over again, then health must be rebuilt the same way. Once you raise your standards for yourself and refuse to accept anything but optimal health, you'll begin to heal. Don't give up on yourself, ever. When your health improves, everything in your life will blossom.

I am here for you. I believe in you. You are powerful. Do everything you can to maximize that power. I am cheering you on.

Recipes

THE FOLLOWING ARE SOME OF my favorite recipes. Many people think that when you eat healthy, your food is going to be tasteless. Nothing could be further from the truth!

I'm sure you'll find the following recipes enjoyable—they will give you sustained energy after you eat or drink them and help make your 45-Day Reset simple and easy to follow.

All ingredients should be bought organic. If you can't find organic versions of a food you want, be sure to follow the EWG's guidelines for the Dirty Dozen and Clean Fifteen, listed in the previous chapter.

These recipes are completely optional. If you don't like to cook, you can keep it really simple and ignore them altogether. I include them because I've noticed that one of the bigger obstacles to long-term success with this style of eating is boredom. The mind likes change, especially when it comes to food. So mix it up, try new smoothies, and when you have time to be adventurous, try a new recipe.

Make it fun and easy for yourself!

Appetizers

SWEET POTATO PANCAKES (4 SERVINGS)

Pretty much everyone grew up eating potato pancakes made from left-over mashed potatoes, but this take on potato pancakes adds a big burst of flavor and health with the use of sweet potatoes, which have far more vitamins, minerals, and flavor than white potatoes. Cooked in coconut oil, they have a slightly sweet yet savory flavor that you'll want to experience again and again.

INGREDIENTS

2 medium sweet potatoes, peeled and shredded

¼ medium onion, shredded

2 large eggs, beaten lightly

1 teaspoon pink Himalayan sea salt

2 tablespoons refined coconut oil

INSTRUCTIONS

Place the first four ingredients in a large mixing bowl. Mix until combined. Heat the coconut oil in a large iron skillet over medium heat, making sure that the pan is fully coated. You might find you need more coconut oil; it's OK to use more, just ensure that the pan is coated. Once the oil is hot, use a ¼-cup measurer to drop the potato mixture into the pan. Press each mound down a little with your spatula. The mounds should look like round pancakes. Fry each pancake until each side is brown and crispy. This should take about four minutes for each side. Avoid turning the pancakes so that they don't come apart. Remove to drain on a paper towel.

Tip: Refined coconut oil can take higher temperatures. For best results, you want the cakes to sizzle when you put them into the pan.

Side Dishes

Butternut Squash with Peas & Parmesan (4 servings)

This is a take on risotto—with all the creamy goodness but without the carbs. But you won't miss the carbs; in fact, you'll wish you had made more of this side dish because your family is going to devour it quickly.

INGREDIENTS

1 butternut squash, peeled and cubed

1 tablespoon avocado oil

1 garlic clove, pressed in a garlic press

¼ teaspoon red pepper flakes

¼ yellow onion, chopped

2 tablespoons vegetable broth

1 cup vegetable broth or bone broth (see recipe below)

¼ cup peas, cooked and drained

¼ cup raw parmesan cheese, grated

Salt and pepper, to taste

INSTRUCTIONS

Rice the squash in a food processor and then save for later. One trick to ricing vegetables successfully is to use a spiralizer first. You can find one on Amazon. Cut off the peel of the butternut squash, spiralize, and then place it in a food processor. Pulse a few times in the food processor and you will have riced butternut squash.

In a small pan over medium heat, warm 1 cup of the vegetable broth; keep ready. In a large skillet, heat the olive oil and add the onion to the pan, cooking to sweat the onions for about 2 minutes. Then add the garlic and red pepper flakes, cooking another 30 seconds. Add the 2 tablespoons of broth and let cook for an additional 2 minutes. Toss in the riced butternut squash plus salt and pepper, stirring gently to combine. Add in half the remaining warm broth, cooking for another few minutes and watching for it to get dry. Then add in the rest of the broth, allowing it to reduce again. Start tasting the squash, and if it's not done, you can keep adding in a little broth at a time until the squash is tender. When squash is tender, add in the peas, stirring carefully to combine and heat through. Add the cheese and stir to melt.

Sweet Potato and Cabbage Slaw (6 servings)
You may not have realized you can eat raw sweet potato, but it's a lot like carrots—only better! This version of slaw will awaken your taste buds, and the added spice will make you super happy and wide awake.

Ingredients

2 tablespoons avocado oil

1 tablespoon lime juice

1-½ teaspoons toasted sesame oil

½ teaspoon pink Himalayan sea salt

3 cups sweet potato, grated

3 cups Napa cabbage, shredded

4 scallions, trimmed and sliced thin

1 teaspoon jalapeno peppers, finely minced

INSTRUCTIONS

In a large bowl, whisk together the oils, lime juice, and salt. Toss in the potato, cabbage, scallions, and peppers. Serve.

Tip: If you want to serve later, don't mix in the sauce until it's time to serve.

SWEET POTATO COINS (4 SERVINGS)

This recipe was born out of a need to create better side dishes that my children would love. Sweet potatoes are lower on the glycemic index than white potatoes. This recipe is easy to make, delicious to eat, and helps reset your health. You can experiment with your favorite spices very easily. Even fresh herbs like basil or oregano can liven it up.

INGREDIENTS
2 to 3 medium-size sweet potatoes, sliced into thin coin shapes
2 tablespoons coconut oil
Himalayan salt, to taste

INSTRUCTIONS

Slice the sweet potatoes into thin rounds. Place in a large mixing bowl and add coconut oil. Make sure that there is enough coconut oil to cover all the sweet potato coins. Sprinkle with Himalayan salt to taste. Lay the coins flat on a cookie sheet, making sure that none of the coins are overlapping each other. Place in the oven on the top rack and put the oven on medium broil. Cook for 10 minutes, keeping a close eye on the coins to make sure they don't brown too quickly. Turn each coin over after 10 minutes and place back in the oven for another 5 minutes. Once crispy, remove. Let cool down and enjoy!

Main Courses

Coconut Chicken Curry Stew (8 servings)

You can't go wrong with this curry stew. You're going to love it all year long because it's not weighed down and heavy. Using coconut milk and filling it out with veggies like zucchini make it super-healthy brain food. Your family will thank you.

Ingredients

2 tablespoons refined coconut oil

8 boneless, skinless, organic chicken thighs, cut into 1-inch pieces

1 large yellow onion, roughly chopped into large chunks

3 small zucchini, thickly sliced

1 teaspoon garlic, minced

1 tablespoon curry powder

½ teaspoon paprika

2 teaspoons course pink Himalayan sea salt

30 ounces unsweetened coconut milk

1 cup red grape tomatoes

Cilantro, optional garnish

INSTRUCTIONS

In a large pot with oil, set on high heat, brown the chicken on both sides. Remove the chicken from the pan and set aside. In the same pan, add the onion, sweat the onion for about 2 minutes, and then add in the zucchini. Sauté both until slightly browned, then add in the garlic, curry, paprika, and salt, and sauté an additional 30 seconds. Put the chicken back in the pot with the ingredients, add in the coconut milk, and bring to a boil. Reduce and simmer, covered, for about 20 minutes or until the chicken is tender and cooked through. Add in the tomatoes and cook an additional 5 or 10 minutes. Serve like stew, with cilantro as garnish if desired.

TEX-MEX LOW-CARB BURRITO BOWL (4 SERVINGS)

Who doesn't like Tex-Mex night? No one, right? Of course, it can be hard on the waistline and belly, but this pared-down version is low carb and full of goodness, with lots of flavor. Eat it in a bowl, top it with extra salsa, and you'll be so happy you did.

INGREDIENTS

2 tablespoons avocado oil

3 cups broccoli slaw

1/3 cup yellow onion, chopped

1/3 cup red bell pepper, chopped

1/3 cup celery, chopped

2 cloves garlic, pressed

1 pound ground grass-fed beef

2 to 4 diced green chilies

1-½ tablespoons chili powder

2 teaspoons ground cumin

Salt and pepper, to taste

Cilantro

Avocado, sliced

INSTRUCTIONS

In a large sauté pan, heat up the avocado oil, add onion, and sweat for 1 minute, stirring continuously. Add the bell pepper, stir for another minute, add the celery and broccoli slaw, sauté for another 2 minutes, and finally add the garlic. Cook, stirring the entire time, until the broccoli slaw is of desired doneness. In another pan, brown the ground beef, drain off, add green chilies, and then add the rest of the spices except for the salt and pepper, cilantro, and avocado. To prepare your burrito bowl, layer the veggies with the meat in a bowl. Top with cilantro and avocado.

Tip: Get creative with your toppings. What can you grow and use? Find your favorites.

ASIAN TURKEY LETTUCE WRAPS (4 SERVINGS)

This is my absolutely favorite main course recipe. My kids love it when we make these—and they can be picky eaters. I prefer the cashew butter for a richer taste. It's easy to make. Enjoy!

INGREDIENTS

1 pound ground organic turkey
1 cup Shitake mushroom caps, chopped
3 tablespoons organic almond or cashew butter
1 tablespoon sesame oil
1 tablespoon rice vinegar
1 8-ounce can water chestnuts, chopped
3 cloves garlic, minced
2 tablespoons fresh ginger, minced
1/3 cup soy sauce
½ cup green onions, chopped
1 head lettuce, separated into leaves (We like butter lettuce.)

INSTRUCTIONS

Cook the turkey in a skillet for about 5 minutes, until the turkey crumbles and is no longer pink. Add the mushrooms and the next 7 ingredients. Cook on medium-high heat, stirring constantly, for 4 minutes. Add green onions if desired and cook 1 minute. Spoon the mixture evenly onto lettuce leaves and roll them up. Serve with extra soy sauce if desired.

From B. J. Hardick, Kimberly Roberto, and Ben Lerner, *Maximized Living Nutrition Plans* (Celebration, FL: Maximized Living, 2009).

GRAINLESS SANDWICH (1 SERVING)

Think you'll never eat a sandwich again? Not necessarily true. There are creative ways in which you can make sandwiches without bread. I like to use romaine lettuce because it's stiff and holds the contents of the sandwich well. I have also used large butter lettuce leaves. Here's one of my favorite lunchtime treats.

INGREDIENTS
2 romaine lettuce leaves (the larger the better)
½ avocado, sliced
2 slices organic no-nitrite deli meat (turkey or chicken preferred)
1 slice tomato
2 slices raw cheese

INSTRUCTIONS

Rinse and then pat dry the lettuce leaves. Put the avocado slices on first. Then add the meat and tomato, followed by the cheese. Roll up like you would a wrap. If the contents start to fall out, wrap a second piece of lettuce around it. If you need more moisture or spice, try adding some Sriracha sauce.

GRASS-FED BURGERS (4 SERVINGS)

This is a recipe that we often make for dinner in my household. I like to have these burgers with a green salad and sweet potato coins on the side. Grass-fed burgers are also great wrapped in large pieces of butter lettuce.

INGREDIENTS
1 pound grass-fed burger meat
¼ red onion, diced
1 teaspoon raw organic butter
1 cup raw organic grated cheese (optional)
Himalayan salt
Ground pepper

INSTRUCTIONS
Heat the butter in a small skillet and add red onions. Cook for 3 to 5 minutes. Don't let the onions blacken. Remove the onions from heat and cool. Put the meat in a separate bowl. Place the cooled onions on top of the meat and mix thoroughly. Add grated cheese. Mix so that the onions and cheese are throughout the entire meat mixture. Add salt and pepper to taste. Form the mixture into patties. Put on a cooking sheet and place in the oven on broil.

Salads

CALIFORNIAN COBB SALAD (4 SERVINGS)

You will find that salads will become a common meal for you. What I love about a salad is that you can get a great combination of good fats, protein, and raw vegetables in one meal. Here is a version of a Cobb salad that I like to make often. Everyone loves the fried egg on top. When you cut it, the yolk will seep into the salad and add to the taste.

INGREDIENTS

3 cups mixed greens

1 cup chopped parsley

2 cups chopped organic turkey or chicken (Sliced uncured meats are OK too.)

½ cup chopped raw cheese

½ avocado, sliced

1 to 4 fried eggs (one for each serving)

1 teaspoon grass-fed butter

INSTRUCTIONS

Wash the mixed greens and place in a large salad bowl. Chop the parsley, meats, and cheese and toss them into the salad. Slice the avocado.

Cook a fried egg in butter on the stovetop. If desired, let the egg yolk be a bit runny. Mix the chopped items into the greens. Toss with salad dressing (see my favorite salad dressing recipe) and put on a large dinner plate. Place avocado slices on top. Then place a fried egg on top of each plate you serve salad on.

GREEN APPLE AND RAW NUT SALAD (4 TO 6 SERVINGS)

I have brought this salad to dinner parties for years and everyone loves it. It's high in protein and lots of good fats. Be sure to use the salad dressing recipe I give you—it really brings out the taste of the green apples.

INGREDIENTS
3 cups organic mixed greens
1 cup mint sprigs
½ cucumber, chopped
2 green apples, thinly sliced
½ cup raw almonds
Salad dressing

INSTRUCTIONS
Wash and rinse the mixed greens. Place them in a large salad bowl. Add mint. Thinly slice the green apples and chop the cucumbers. Toss the items into bowls with the greens. Toss in almonds (no need to chop). Right before serving, add dressing for best taste. Feel free to add chopped meats or cheese for more protein and healthy fats.

Breakfast Salad (1 serving)

The most common question I get from patients is "What do I eat for breakfast?" With your 45-day program you will have to think outside the box a bit. A breakfast salad is a great way to start your day off healthy. This is quick and easy, and it will give you lots of energy to start your day.

Ingredients
1 cup organic mixed greens
1 avocado, sliced
½ cup raw nuts
1 fried egg
1 teaspoon grass-fed butter

Instructions

After you wash and dry the mixed greens, place them on a plate. Fry an egg in a pan with grass-fed butter. Cook to your desired yolk firmness. Cut the avocado and place on the greens on a plate. Place almonds on top of that. Finish with a fried egg on top. Salad dressing optional, but I usually don't put salad dressing on this one, making for one less step in the morning. Enjoy!

Reset Factor Salad Dressing (4 to 6 servings)

Commercial salad dressing is packed with sugar and chemicals. You want to avoid it at all costs. I discovered this homemade salad dressing years ago, and I get a ton of comments on it every time I bring a salad over to someone's house for dinner. I also love how easy it is to make.

INGREDIENTS
1 lemon
1 cup olive oil
1 tablespoon fig jam (without sugar, fruit only)

INSTRUCTIONS
Put the oil in a bowl. Squeeze the lemon in, removing seeds. Stir in the jam. Mix thoroughly so there are no chunks of jam left. I have used many different versions of jam. Apricot is good as well. You can also use stevia instead of jam if you are on the 15-Day Detox.

Soups and Stews

HEARTY LAMB STEW (4 SERVINGS)
When we want to warm up in our house, this is our go-to food. We try to make the batch last two to three days. Local farmers' markets are great locations to find new ingredients to add.

INGREDIENTS
2 tablespoons avocado oil
3 pounds grass-fed lamb stew meat, with bone (Have the butcher cut it for you.)
1 cup red onion, chopped
1/3 cup celery, chopped
2 cloves garlic, chopped
2 tablespoons ground Garam Masala spice blend
1-½ cups shitake mushrooms, chopped
2 sweet potatoes or yams, chopped
2 lemons or limes, juiced or squeezed
3 cups beef or lamb bone broth (see recipe)
Salt and pepper to taste

Instructions

Using a large bowl, cover the lamb with 1 tablespoon of avocado oil and then the spice mix. Add more spice as needed so as to cover all sides of the meat. In a large soup pot, heat up the remaining avocado oil on high, add onion, and sweat for 1 minute, stirring continuously. Add the spiced lamb and celery, and finally add in the garlic. Cook, stirring frequently to prevent burning. When the meat has an even sear, add 1 cup of broth as well as the sweet potatoes and mushrooms. Then add a second cup of broth. Bring this to a boil, then turn the heat to medium-low and cover. Stir frequently to keep the flavors combined. Add in the citrus juice. The sweet potatoes should dissolve as the stew cooks. Add the last cup of broth and simmer for at least half an hour before serving. Spice to taste. Remember to store the soup in the refrigerator when it's not on the stove. Add broth and ingredients to keep the pot going, as the base will get better and better.

Spa Soup (8 to 10 servings)

In my family, we call this one spa soup because it's like a spa for your digestive system. We often cook this delicious soup the day after Christmas, when everyone has overeaten and needs a good reset to their gut.

Ingredients

1-¼ pounds sweet potatoes

1-½ teaspoons sea salt

2 to 3 tablespoons fresh sage leaves, chopped

1 bunch Russian kale (8 ounces)

1 bunch green chard (8 ounces)

8 cloves garlic, peeled

3 cups vegetable broth

---

2 large yellow onions
2 tablespoons avocado oil
Freshly ground black pepper
Fresh lemon juice

INSTRUCTIONS

Peel and dice the sweet potatoes. Combine them in a large soup pot with 3-½ cups water, a teaspoon of salt, and the sage. Bring to a boil, then lower the heat and simmer, covered, for about 10 minutes. Wash the kale and chard, trimming away the tough stems. Chop the greens coarsely. Add the greens to the soup, along with the garlic cloves and the vegetable broth. Continue simmering gently, covered, for another 20 minutes.

Meanwhile, chop the onions and sauté them gently with a pinch of sea salt in avocado oil on the stovetop over medium heat. Stir frequently, until they are soft and golden brown, for 30 to 40 minutes. When the onions are ready, add them to the soup and let it cool slightly. Puree the soup in a blender, in batches, and return it to a clean pot. Add a little more water or broth if the soup is too thick to pour easily from a ladle. Serve hot. Squeeze lemon on top and add black pepper for added taste.

Probiotic Rich Foods

Probiotic Yogurt (10 to 12 servings)

Making your own yogurt from raw dairy can be a great way to get probiotics into your diet. Unlike pasteurized yogurt, homemade raw yogurt will have multiple strains of good probiotics and will benefit your gut greatly. Here is a simple recipe you can follow to make your own yogurt. There are three steps:

Step 1: Start with raw organic whole milk.

Step 2: Purchase a probiotic starter online. There are lots of great options on Amazon.

Step 3: Make your delicious yogurt!

Instructions

Heat the milk on the stovetop to 180 degrees, stirring constantly. This breaks down proteins. Once the milk is thick, remove it from heat and let it cool down to 110 degrees. Once it's at a 110 degrees, add the probiotic mix into the milk. Pour into mason jars and put in the refrigerator for 8 to 10 hours. One trick to make this quick and easy is to buy an electric yogurt maker, which maintains the temperature and assures that you get the best finished yogurt possible.

SAUERKRAUT (10 TO 12 SERVINGS)

Sauerkraut is one of the best probiotic-rich foods that you can eat. It literally has trillions of good bacteria in it. Many experts feel that you will get more probiotics from eating sauerkraut than you will from taking a probiotic. Here's how you make it.

INGREDIENTS

2 large cabbages (Reserve 3 to 4 large leaves, enough to cover the surface of the brewing container.)

2 large onions (You can use other vegetables as well—hot peppers, carrots, beets, caraway seeds, ginger, and garlic also make your sauerkraut great!)

2 teaspoons sea salt

1 cup filtered water

1 cup apple cider vinegar

INSTRUCTIONS

Shred the cabbage and other vegetables in a food processor. Put the shredded vegetables in a large container with all the other ingredients. Pound them with a mallet or pestle—long enough to release the juices. Press the mash down. The juices should just about cover the top of the mash. Put a large plate on top of the mash to help release more of the juices. Leave on countertop for a couple of hours. Within a few hours, liquids should cover the tip of the shredded mixture. If there is not enough cabbage juice, add cold filtered water or more apple cider vinegar. Leave to ferment at room temperature for 3 to 5 days. Within 1 day the smell should start to change, and within 3 days the mixture should have a delicious aroma. Transfer to jars and place in the refrigerator. The longer your sauerkraut stays in your refrigerator, the more great bacteria it will create.

Bone Broth (10 to 12 servings)

If you think you have leaky gut syndrome, consuming bone broth is one of the best ways to heal and seal those microholes. If you think you have a severe leaky gut condition, do a bone broth fast for four days, then add in high-probiotic foods like sauerkraut and probiotic yogurt. The bone broth will repair microholes and kill bad bacteria. The sauerkraut and yogurt will add trillions of new good bacteria to your gut. It's a great way to reset your gut.

In selecting the bones for the broth, look for high-quality bones from grass-fed beef, bison, pastured organic poultry, or wild-caught fish. Since you will be extracting the minerals and drinking them in concentrated form, you want to make sure that the animal was as healthy as possible.

There are several places to obtain good bones for stock:

- Save leftovers from when you roast a chicken, duck, or turkey (organic and pasture raised)
- From a local butcher, especially one who butchers the whole animal
- From a local farmer who raises grass-fed animals (ask around at your local farmers' market)
- Online from companies like US Wellness Meats or Tropical Traditions

---

Ingredients

2 pounds (or more) bones from a healthy source (This is about 2 to 3 chickens.)

2 chicken feet for extra gelatin (optional)

1 onion

2 carrots

3 stalks celery

3 tubers turmeric (optional)

2 tablespoons apple cider vinegar

Optional:
1 bunch parsley
1 tablespoon or more sea salt
1 teaspoon peppercorns
Additional herbs and spices
2 cloves garlic (add for the last 30 minutes of cooking for additional taste)

INSTRUCTIONS

Place the ingredients in a large stock pot on the stovetop. I like to put my bone broth in a slow cooker—either way works. Add enough water to cover the bones. Place on medium to high heat for several hours. Within the first hour, a foam will develop on the top. Scoop that foam off. After several hours, put the broth on low heat and cook for 24 to 48 hours. The apple cider vinegar will pull many nutrients and minerals out of the bones. After several days, you can strain the bones and vegetables and serve the broth. I leave it in my slow cooker and scoop the broth out. Then I keep adding more water to extend the broth.

Desserts

Chocolate Coconut Bars (8 servings)

Just because you've pulled sugar out of your diet doesn't mean that you have to be deprived of sweets. Who doesn't love chocolate and coconut? These bars will satisfy your sweet tooth and give you healthy fats.

INGREDIENTS

Bottom Layer

2 cups shredded coconut, unsweetened

1/3 cup virgin coconut oil, melted

2 droppers liquid stevia

Top Layer

3 squares unsweetened baker's chocolate

1 tablespoon coconut oil

2 droppers liquid stevia

INSTRUCTIONS

To prepare the bottom layer, place all the ingredients in a food processor with the S blade and blend the ingredients until dough is formed.

Scrape the sides as needed. Press into a cold 8 x 8 silicon cake pan and place in the freezer. To prepare the top layer, using a medium to small glass bowl, warm the coconut oil and baker's chocolate on low on the stovetop. When melted, stir in the sweetener. Remove the bottom layer from the freezer and spread chocolate evenly over the bottom layer. Freeze for 30 minutes.

Tip: Spread toasted almond slivers between layers for an added kick of protein and flavor.

Grain-Free Cookies (6 to 12 servings)

You might think that going grain-free means you'll never eat a cookie again, but nothing is further from the truth. Here are some great dessert options that will satisfy your taste buds without raising your insulin levels.

Ingredients
1 cup super-chunky peanut butter (½ cup almond butter or peanut butter)
1 cup coconut sugar
1 large egg
1 teaspoon baking soda
½ teaspoon vanilla extract
1 cup miniature semisweet chocolate chips (about 6 ounces) (I recommend Lillie's Stevia Sweetened Chocolate Chips, available at Whole Foods.)

INSTRUCTIONS

Preheat oven to 350 degrees. Mix the first 5 ingredients in a medium bowl. Mix in the chocolate chips. Using moistened hands, form a generous tablespoon of dough for each cookie into a ball (flatten the ball once on the pan). Arrange them on 2 ungreased baking sheets, spacing 2 inches apart. Bake cookies until puffed, golden on the bottom and still soft to touch in the center, for about 12 minutes. Cool on sheets for 5 minutes. Transfer to racks; cool completely.

ALMOND CHOCOLATE POWER BARS (8 TO 10 SERVINGS)

There is no doubt that this is one of my favorite dessert recipes. It's easy to make (prep time is 8 minutes and cooking time is 12), helps satisfy a nighttime sweet tooth, and is packed with so many good fats that it helps to stabilize your blood sugar for days. I often have a container of these at the office to snack on throughout the day to keep my energy high.

INGREDIENTS

2 cups raw almonds
½ cup flaxseed meal
½ cup unsweetened shredded coconut
2 scoops flavored whey protein powder
½ cup raw almond butter
½ teaspoon kosher salt
½ cup coconut oil
8 drops liquid stevia or ¾ teaspoon stevia powder, to taste
1 tablespoon pure vanilla extract (no sugar—check the label)
8 squares unsweetened chocolate, melted and sweetened to taste with stevia and cinnamon (optional)

INSTRUCTIONS

Place the almonds, flax meal, shredded coconut, whey powder, almond butter, and salt in a food processor. Pulse briefly, for about 10 seconds. In a small saucepan, melt the coconut oil over very low heat. Remove the coconut oil from the stove, then stir the stevia and vanilla into the oil. Add the coconut oil mixture to a food processor and pulse until the ingredients from a coarse paste. Press the mixture into an 8 x 8 glass baking dish. (A parchment paper liner helps when you want to remove the bars from the dish.) Chill in the refrigerator for 1 hour, until the mixture hardens. In a double boiler, melt the chocolate, stirring in stevia and cinnamon. Spread melted chocolate over the bars and return to the refrigerator for 30 minutes, until the chocolate hardens. Remove from the refrigerator, cut into bars, and serve.

Adapted from B. J. Hardick, Kimberly Roberto, and Ben Lerner, *Maximized Living Nutrition Plans* (Celebration, FL: Maximized Living, 2009).

Breakfast

Pesto Chicken and Sweet Potato Breakfast Bake (4 servings)

Here's a great Sunday morning brunch option. Packed with lots of good fats and clean proteins, this breakfast should keep you full and energized for hours.

INGREDIENTS

4 tablespoons melted ghee, butter, or coconut oil, divided into equal parts

1 small sweet potato, peeled and diced

½ yellow onion, minced

2 garlic cloves, minced

2 cups diced cooked chicken (I use a rotisserie chicken.)

3 tablespoons homemade pesto (or you can just use fresh basil)

10 eggs, whisked

Salt, to taste

INSTRUCTIONS

Preheat oven to 400 degrees. Toss the sweet potatoes in 2 tablespoons of ghee. Place on a parchment paper on a lined baking sheet and bake for 25 to 30 minutes until soft, then turn oven temperature down to 350 degrees. Place a large sauté pan over medium heat and add 2 more tablespoons of ghee along with the onion and garlic. Cook until the onions become translucent, about 5 minutes. Add the chicken and cook for about 10 minutes. Last, add pesto and mix well until combined. Grease an 8 x 8 baking dish, add the mixture from the pan to the baking dish, and then add in eggs and salt along with the sweet potatoes. Mix well until combined. Place in the oven and bake for 30 to 35 minutes, until the eggs are set in the middle and cooked through.

Breakfast on the Go: Sausage Egg Cups (4 servings)

I love this quick breakfast option—it's another great way to start your day with a high-protein meal that will keep your blood sugar up all day long.

INGREDIENTS

2 to 3 chicken sausages (hormone- and antibiotic-free), cooked and chopped

1 red bell pepper, chopped

¼ yellow onion, chopped

8 eggs, whisked

2 garlic cloves, minced

¼ teaspoon garlic powder

1/8 teaspoon red pepper flakes

Salt and pepper, to taste

Avocado, to garnish

INSTRUCTIONS

Preheat oven to 325 degrees. Cook the sausage until cooked through. In a large bowl, add the sausage, red bell pepper, yellow onion, eggs, garlic cloves, garlic powder, red pepper flakes, and salt and pepper. Whisk until well combined. Use a ladle to pour the mixture into 8 to 10 muffin tins. (I use a silicone muffin tray and do not have to grease it. If you're using a regular metal pan, thoroughly grease all of it or use muffin liners.) Place in the oven and bake for 35 to 40 minutes or until cooked through. Garnish with avocado.

EASY SPIN ON BREAKFAST (1 TO 2 SERVINGS)

This is another tasty and quick breakfast option. I find that many people don't know what to do for breakfast if they take grains and cereal out of their diet, but eating sweet potatoes is a great way to fill yourself up in the morning.

INGREDIENTS

1 sweet potato or yam, poked with a fork

2 eggs, cooked to preference

For the pesto

2/3 cup walnuts

1 to 1-½ cups fresh basil leaves

1 garlic clove, peeled

½ cup olive oil

juice of ½ lemon

Salt and pepper, to taste

INSTRUCTIONS

Poke holes in the sweet potato with a fork. Wrap the sweet potato in foil and place it in a slow cooker for 8 hours on low or 4 hours on high. To cook faster, place the sweet potato in an oven at 400 degrees for 25 to 35 minutes. Once the sweet potato is done, remove it from the foil to let it cool to the touch before removing the skin. Then mash the sweet potato with a fork. For the pesto, place the walnuts in the food processor along with the basil leaves and garlic clove, and pulse until the leaves break down. Then slowly add the olive oil while the food processor is still running. Lastly, add lemon juice and a bit of salt and pepper. Puree until smooth. Once the sweet potato is mashed and the pesto is finished, mix 2 to 4 tablespoons of the pesto into the mashed sweet potato. To finish off the meal, cook up an egg however you like. I fry mine over easy.

5-INGREDIENT BREAKFAST STUFFED ACORN SQUASH (2 SERVINGS)
If you haven't tried acorn squash, now's a great time. Sweet and with a nice soft texture, this meal could be served for breakfast or dinner.

INGREDIENTS
¾ pound natural breakfast sausage
1 acorn squash, cut in half with seeds removed
2 eggs
½ yellow onion, diced
1 garlic clove, minced
Salt and pepper, to taste

INSTRUCTIONS

Preheat oven to 375 degrees. Place the acorn squash cut-side down onto your baking sheet. Bake for 20 to 25 minutes or until the acorn squash is soft when you press on the skin. Remove it from the oven and let cool. While your acorn squash is cooking, add a tablespoon of some kind of fat to a large pan over medium heat (I use bacon fat), then add your minced garlic and diced onion. Stir to keep from burning. Once your onions become translucent, add your breakfast sausage to the pan. Cook down, breaking up the breakfast sausage as it cooks.

Once the breakfast sausage is almost all the way cooked through, turn your heat to low and add the inside of your acorn squash. Do this by using a spoon to scoop out the insides, leaving just the skin of the acorn squash. Be careful not the tear the skin! Mix the acorn squash and the breakfast sausage together, then add it back to your acorn squash skin. Once both of your acorn squash halves are full, press into the middle with a spoon to create a little resting spot for your egg. Crack an egg on top. Place back in the oven to cook for 10 to 15 minutes or until your egg is cooked to your preference. Serve!

15-Day Detox Smoothies

Very Berry Breakfast (2 servings)

INGREDIENTS
1 cup frozen unsweetened or fresh raspberries
¾ cup chilled unsweetened almond milk
¼ cup frozen pitted or fresh unsweetened cherries or raspberries
2 teaspoons finely grated fresh ginger
1 teaspoon ground flaxseed or flaxseed oil
2 teaspoons fresh lemon juice

INSTRUCTIONS
Pour the milk into a blender. Then add the berries, cherries, and ginger. Mix on high for 1 minute. Then add the grated ginger and lemon juice. Mix on high for another minute.

Berry Good Workout Smoothie (1 serving)

INGREDIENTS
1-½ cups chopped frozen or fresh strawberries
1 cup frozen or fresh blueberries
½ cup frozen or fresh raspberries
1 cup coconut milk
1 teaspoon fresh lemon juice
1 scoop plant or grass-fed whey protein powder
½ cup ice cubes

INSTRUCTIONS
Combine all ingredients in a blender, adding lemon juice to taste. Puree until smooth.

Spinach Smoothie with Avocado and Apple (1 to 2 servings)

INGREDIENTS
1-½ cups coconut milk
2 cups stemmed and chopped spinach or kale
1 green apple—unpeeled and cored
½ avocado, chopped
1 scoop plant or grass-fed whey protein powder
1 cup ice

INSTRUCTIONS

Combine the coconut milk, spinach, apple, and avocado in a blender and puree until smooth, about 1 minute, adding water to reach the desired consistency. Add ice to thicken.

RESET GREEN DETOX SMOOTHIE 1 (1 TO 2 SERVINGS)

INGREDIENTS
3 to 4 cups water
1 avocado
6 stalks collard greens
¼ cup hemp seeds
1 juice of a lemon plus zest (or lime would be fine)
Drops of stevia to taste
1 spoonful sunflower lecithin or almond butter (optional, but we love it as it really helps bind and make smoothies really smooth)
½ teaspoon turmeric (for reducing inflammation—fresh is best)
1 cup ice

INSTRUCTIONS

Pour the water into a blender. Add greens, hemp seeds, lemon, turmeric, and almond butter. Mix on high for 1 minute. Add ice. Mix for another minute. Add stevia to sweeten as needed.

RESET GREEN SMOOTHIE 2 (1 TO 2 SERVINGS)

INGREDIENTS
3 to 4 cups water
1 avocado
4 large handfuls kale (We like to de-stem ours.)
1 handful fresh spinach
Juice and zest of 1 lemon
Drops of stevia to taste
1 inch fresh peeled ginger (sometimes more, as we just love it)
1 spoonful sunflower lecithin or almond butter (optional)
1 tablespoon Udo's omega oil blend (great for brainpower)
1 cup ice

RESET GREEN DETOX SMOOTHIE 3 (1 TO 2 SERVINGS)

INGREDIENTS
3 to 4 cups water
1 avocado
6 stalks collard greens
Handful parsley leaves
Juice and zest of 1 lemon
½ teaspoon turmeric (again, for controlling our inflammation—fresh is best)
1 teaspoon cinnamon

2 tablespoons hemp oil
2 teaspoons sunflower lecithin
Stevia to taste
1 cup ice

INSTRUCTIONS

Place the water and hemp oil in the blender. Then add the avocado, collard greens, parsley, and turmeric. Mix for 1 minute on high. Then add the sunflower lecithin, lemon and zest, and cinnamon. Add ice for a better taste. Add stevia if you need to sweeten. Mix on high for 1 more minute.

MORNING DETOX WATER (1 SERVING)

This is a great way to start your day off right. I recommend that you have this first thing in the morning, as you want the first thing that hits your stomach to be healthy. This morning detox water will help your body be more alkaline, pull mucus from your body, cleanse your liver, and speed up your metabolism. Make this a part of your morning ritual and watch your health grow.

INGREDIENTS
1 pint-size glass of water (about 1 to 2 cups)
1 tablespoon of apple cider vinegar (I like Bragg's.)
1 whole lemon
Dash of cayenne pepper
Dash of cinnamon
Stevia as needed
Grated ginger (optional)

INSTRUCTIONS

Mix all the ingredients in a glass of water. I use a pint glass. You can mix with a spoon or use a blender for best results. When squeezing the lemon in, be sure to take the seeds out. If mornings are tough for you, it's a good idea to make a larger batch to keep in the refrigerator so it's ready to go for the morning.

30-Day Habit Reset Smoothies

Green Tea Smoothie (1 to 2 servings)
Antioxidant-rich green tea makes this smoothie a nutritional powerhouse.

Ingredients
3 tablespoons water
1 green tea bag
2 teaspoons honey
1-½ cups frozen or fresh blueberries
½ medium banana
¾ cup almond milk
1 cup ice

Instructions
Heat the water on high until it's steaming hot in a small bowl. Add the tea bag and allow to brew for 3 minutes. Remove the tea bag. Stir the honey into the tea until it dissolves. Combine the berries, banana, and milk in a blender that has ice-crushing ability. Add the tea to the blender. Blend the ingredients on "Ice Crush" or the highest setting until smooth. (Some blenders may require additional water to process the mixture.) Pour the smoothie into a tall glass and serve.

Watermelon Wonder Smoothie (2 servings)

Transform a summer fruit favorite into a drinkable delight. Just remember to buy seedless watermelon or remove the seeds before you blend!

Ingredients
2 cups chopped watermelon
¼ cup coconut milk
1 tablespoon coconut oil
2 cups ice

Instructions
Combine the watermelon and coconut milk, and blend for 15 seconds or until smooth. Add the ice and blend 20 seconds longer, or to your desired consistency. Add more ice, if needed, and blend for 10 seconds.

Collard Greens Smoothie with Mango and Lime (1 to 2 servings)

Ingredients
2 tablespoons fresh lime juice
2 cups stemmed and chopped collard greens or spinach
1-½ cups frozen mango
1 cup green grapes (freeze ahead for best results)
1 cup ice

INSTRUCTIONS

Combine the lime juice, ½ cup water, collard greens, mango, and grapes in a blender and puree until smooth, about 1 minute, adding more water to reach the desired consistency.

TURMERIC TORNADO SMOOTHIE (1 TO 2 SERVINGS)

Turmeric is a great source of curcumin, which is an anti-inflammatory, antioxidant, anti-tumor, antibacterial, and antiviral agent. It also helps flush out dietary carcinogens, boosts liver detox, and treats depression.

INGREDIENTS

1 cup hemp or coconut milk
½ cup frozen pineapple or mango chunks
1 fresh banana
1 tablespoon coconut oil
½ teaspoon turmeric (can be increased to 1 teaspoon)
½ teaspoon cinnamon
½ teaspoon ginger
1 teaspoon chia seeds
1 teaspoon maca powder (optional)
1 cup ice

INSTRUCTIONS

Process these ingredients in a blender until smooth and enjoy the multiple benefits of turmeric.

About the Author

DR. MINDY PELZ HAS BEEN serving health to her community for over twenty years. After receiving an undergraduate degree in exercise physiology and nutrition from the University of Kansas, she went on to get her doctorate in chiropractic from Palmer West College of Chiropractic, where she graduated with clinical honors.

Dr. Mindy knows what it's like to have your health taken from you. At a young age, she was diagnosed with chronic fatigue syndrome (CFS) and told to drop out of school and wait for medication to work. Refusing to believe the prognosis the doctors gave her, she went searching for answers. Her personal journey back to health ignited a voracious passion in her to understand why the human body breaks down—and how these breakdowns can be fixed by removing toxins, adding in good nutrition, and working with the healing laws of the body.

In the 20 years she has been in practice, Dr. Mindy has helped tens of thousands of people reset their health. Her unique approach to health and her passion for nutrition has led her to work with professionals, Olympic and collegiate athletes, Academy Award–winning actors, professional musicians, and Silicon Valley CEOs. She lectures all over the country and has been hired by numerous corporations to help their employees reduce stress, maximize their nutrition, and remove harmful toxins from their life so they can be healthier, happier, more productive people.

Raising a family of her own, Dr. Mindy is deeply concerned about the toxic world our children are growing up in today and the breakdown many women are experiencing in their perimenopausal years. Dr. Mindy believes that healthy adults start with healthy children. In her own practice, she works closely with all members of many families to give them a toolset to steer their health in whatever direction they choose. The principles she teaches empower every family member to be the boss of their own health and give them a path to predictable health—free of disease, drugs, and surgeries.

Still maintaining an active wellness practice, Dr. Mindy lives in Silicon Valley with her husband and two teenage kids.

Made in the USA
Monee, IL
14 May 2023